Acute Pulmonary Insufficiency

# Acute Pulmonary Insufficiency

## The Role of Haemostatic, Fibrinolytic and Related Mechanisms

Edited by
Tom Saldeen

W DE G
Walter de Gruyter
Berlin · New York 1985

*Editor*

Prof. Tom Saldeen, M. D., Ph. D.
Institute of Forensic Medicine
University of Uppsala
Dag Hammarskjölds Väg 17-19
S-752 37 Uppsala

This book contains 62 illustrations and 10 tables.

*CIP-Kurztitelaufnahme der Deutschen Bibliothek*

**Acute pulmonary insufficiency** : the role of haemostat., fibrinolyt. and related mechanisms / ed. by Tom Saldeen. - Berlin ; New York : de Gruyter, 1985.
ISBN 3-11-010567-5 (Berlin)
ISBN 0-89925-080-7 (New York)
NE: Saldeen, Tom [Hrsg.]

*Library of Congress Cataloging in Publication Data*

Acute pulmonary insufficiency.
Based on a conference on „Post-traumatic organ insufficiency--role of haemostatic, fibrinolytic and related mechanisms, „held during the IXth Congress of the International Society on Thrombosis and Haemostatis, in Stockholm, 1983.
Includes bibliographies.
1. Respiratory distress syndrome, Adult--Congresses.
2. Hemostatis--Congresses. 3. Fibrinolysis--Congresses.
I. Saldeen, Tom. II. International Congress on Thrombosis and Haemostasis (9th : 1983 : Stockholm, Sweden) III. Title: Post-traumatic organ insufficiency--role of haemostatic, fibrinolytic, and related mechanisms. [DNLM: 1. Respiratory Distress Syndrome, Adult--congresses. 2. Wounds and Injuries--complications--congresses. WF 140 A1834)] RC775.R38A279 1985 616.2'4 85-15861
ISBN 0-89925-080-7

ISBN 3 11 010567 5 Walter de Gruyter · Berlin · New York
ISBN 0-89925-080-7 Walter de Gruyter, Inc., Berlin · New York

 Printing: Gerike GmbH, Berlin. - Binding: Dieter Mikolai, Berlin. - Cover design: Rudolf Hübler. - Printed in Germany.

# PREFACE

During the IXth Congress of the International Society on Thrombosis and Haemostasis in Stockholm, 1983, a conference on "Post-traumatic organ insufficiency - Role of haemostatic, fibrinolytic and related mechanisms" was arranged. Some of the papers delivered at this conference concerned acute pulmonary insufficiency. The authors of these papers were later asked to contribute to this book.

Acute pulmonary insufficiency (the adult respiratory distress syndrome) is a common and serious complication following trauma and in connection with sepsis. It is estimated that in the United States 150,000 patients suffer from this syndrome every year and that the mortality is 40 - 50 per cent. It has been recognized for a long time that this syndrome is associated with disturbances in the haemostatic and fibrinolytic systems as well as other related systems. Factors putatively implicated in the pathogenesis include fibrin, fibrin degradation products, platelets, leucocytes, bradykinin and thromboxane. Heparin, dextran, corticosteroids and cyclooxygenase inhibitors have been tried, among other drugs, in the prophylaxis and treatment of this condition. This book consists of reviews of recent work and the present knowledge concerning the role of haemostatic, fibrinolytic and other related mechanisms in acute pulmonary insufficiency.

The book has been sponsored by the Swedish government.

My special thanks are due to Mrs Vera Inglis for skilled secretarial assistance.

Tom Saldeen

# CONTENTS

# BLOOD ALTERATIONS IN THE ADULT RESPIRATORY DISTRESS SYNDROME

ANGELINA C.A. CARVALHO, M.D. AND
WARREN M. ZAPOL, M.D.

Hematology Section, Veterans Administration Medical Center, Brown University, Providence, Rhode Island, USA

and

Massachusetts General Hospital and Harvard Medical School, Boston, Massachusetts, USA

# I. INTRODUCTION

Adult respiratory distress (ARDS) is a complex syndrome which commonly follows septicemia, trauma, severe viral and bacterial respiratory infection, acute abdominal catastrophes, drug intoxication, gastric aspiration, and many other lung insults. This disorder often affects young and previously healthy individuals and is associated with excessive mortality. It is estimated that every year over 150,000 hospitalized Americans develop ARDS and one-half of them succumb to it (16, 31, 38).

Although various factors can cause acute pulmonary injury, the outcome is a predictable sequence of pulmonary pathologic findings which include edema, hemorrhage, hyaline membrane formation, micro- and macrothrombi, inflammatory cells, and fibrosis (36, 51).

Deranged hemostasis has been reported to occur in association with acute lung injury for as long as the syndrome has been recognized; however, the precise nature of the relationship of hemostasis and lung injury remains unclear. We do not know which of the etiologies of ARDS manifest as a coagulopathy that precedes and may cause pulmonary injury, and which are characterized by a coagulopathy that follows the lung injury and perhaps compounds it. We do know, however, that the same diverse factors listed as etiologies of ARDS also cause intravascular coagulation (thrombosis of the microcirculation) with fibrinolysis (50), a syndrome that almost always accompanies ARDS but can occur in its absence.

In this review, we intend to discuss the possible pathways by which blood-borne serine proteases, e.g., thrombin, plasmin, kallikrein, and other mediators released by activated platelets and leukocytes, may act upon pulmonary endothelium to produce injury and promote pulmonary edema.

First, we shall review briefly several current concepts of the pathogenesis of ARDS and then selectively review current concepts of deranged hemostasis in this syndrome.

# II. PATHOGENESIS OF ARDS

## A. Acute lung injury

The sequence of events leading to ARDS begins with injury to the pulmonary endothelium or alveolar epithelium. As a result of such injury, permeability is altered in the pulmonary capillaries, in the alveolar epithelial cells, or in both. This increased permeability leads to excessive loss of water and solutes from the pulmonary capillary bed initially at normal and later at raised pulmonary capillary pressures. Water and solutes accumulate in the interstitial space, in swollen lung cells, in the alveoli, and often in the airways. The edematous fluid that leaks across the injured endothelium typically contains high concentrations of protein. The proteins in edema fluids are in equilibrium with plasma proteins. In severe injury to lung issue, the formed elements of the blood are liberated into the interstitial and intraalveolar spaces. The exudate produces an inflammatory reaction with major secondary changes in the lung's interstitial space, pulmonary capillaries, and alveolar epithelium. The diagnosis of ARDS is usually delayed because considerable endothelial damage must occur before pulmonary edema can be clinically diagnosed.

Atelectasis is prominent in ARDS. Alterations of pulmonary surfactant may be involved in the pathogenesis of atelactasis during ARDS (23). Under normal circumstances, surfactant maintains relatively low surface tension at the air/liquid interspaces of the lung. Abnormal surfactant leads to a high surface tension with resultant alveolar instability and collapse. Thus, the resolution of ARDS is slow and often incomplete. Substantial time is required for restoration of capillary integrity and, in many instances, it does not occur. Recovery is thus complicated by the profound inflammatory process which represents an important component of this syndrome.

The critical issue in the pathogenesis of ARDS is to determine the mechanisms which cause pulmonary endothelial damage and protein-rich capillary leakage.

## B. Blood alterations in ARDS

The findings of a common pulmonary pathological response pattern to the various insults causing ARDS has encouraged a search for the common denominator of pulmonary endothelial injury. The common denominator has been postulated to be a decreased intracellular respiration rate, resulting in ATP levels insufficient to sustain normal endothelial cell function (60). Although reduced cellular respiration is the final concomitant of cell death, it remains unclear how cells become deprived of their nutrients and oxygen. Does fibrin, clogged in the microcirculation, incite pulmonary endothelial injury? Three pioneers in the study of acute lung injury (8, 58) have proposed thromboembolism as a principal etiologic factor of ARDS Studying patients after trauma, Saldeen has postulated that activation of the blood coagulation system occurs at the region of injury and that fibrin-microthrombi, formed in the systemic circulation, are trapped in the lung. Fibrin and its derivatives are noxious agents in the lung and are responsible for endothelial swelling and increased capillary permeability (58,59). Saldeen has described certain types of posttraumatic ARDS as the "pulmonary microembolism syndrome". There is considerable clinical evidence that pulmonary thromboemboli are frequent in ARDS (22, 29, 69) and are associated with a high mortality rate (22).

Acute disseminated intravascular coagulation has been reported in ARDS by several investigators, although they have reported different rates of incidence (9, 13, 22, 64). Elevated fibrin-(ogen) degradation product levels have been found in the blood of ARDS patients (39). Fragment D has been proposed as a marker and mediator of pulmonary microvascular injury (27).

Clinical observations of blood coagulation alterations in ARDS have prompted several investigators to test the hypothesis that *in vivo* induction of microthrombosis may cause acute pulmonary injury. There is substantial experimental evidence in laboratory animals suggesting that both particulate and soluble products of intravascular coagulation and fibrinolysis can cause pulmonary microvascular injury (2, 40, 41, 43, 57). Saturation of the reticuloendothelial system, the latter being an important mechanism for clearing intravascular fibrin, by fibrin(ogen) degradation products and injured platelets, results in augmentation of pulmonary edema and an increased pulmonary artery pressure after the intravenous injection of thrombin (65).

Several inciting factors to activation of blood coagulation in ARDS patients have been inferred from clinical and experimental studies. Release of tissue factors at sites of traumatic injury in ARDS patients was the first pathway proposed for intravascular coagulation in post-traumatic ARDS (8, 58). Platelet activation followed by platelet microaggregates lodging in the lung's microcirculation was reported by Berman in 1969. He believed tissue thrombin caused platelet microaggregate formation and that filtered platelets were sequestered by the lung causing acute pulmonary injury. The studies of Manwaring and Curreri (1983) suggest that fibrinolysis can potentiate consumption in ARDS and mediate pulmonary edema. In patients with septicemia, platelets may be directly activated by endotoxin binding to a specific platelet membrane receptor, followed by platelet content leakage and unmasking of platelet-membrane procoagulants (26). More recently, complement and leukocyte-mediated injury in the alveolus (48,67) or in the systemic circulation (17, 24) has been suggested to cause intravascular coagulation (Hageman factor activation) and lung injury. Although experimental data suggest that products of activated blood coagulation and mediators released by platelets and leukocytes can produce pulmonary endothelial injury, a causal relationship in ARDS patients is difficult to prove. Primary pulmonary endothelial injury can activate both platelets and blood coagulation and this is considered to be the usual pathway by which blood changes occur in ARDS. We should consider, however, that the reverse process may also play a role.

## HEMOSTATIC DEFECTS IN ARDS

The literature described blood changes associated with ARDS which can best be summarized by looking first at the hemostatic defects of patients who suffered major traumatic injury and then at the defects of those who did not suffer traumatic injury.

### A. The hemostatic defect in post-traumatic ARDS

#### 1. Intravascular coagulation with fibrinolysis. (ICF)

Intravascular coagulation with fibrinolysis is one of the most common blood alterations found in ARDS patients after major trauma. The laboratory abnormalities that have been reported are a prolonged prothrombin time, reduced factor VII (29), reduced platelet count and fibrinogen concentration, shortened $^{125}$I-fibrinogen survival time, enhanced fibrinogen turnover rate, and elevated FDP level (22, 29, 58, 64). These blood changes are consistent with the diagnosis of ICF. Clinically, when patients with moderate and severe ARDS had lung biopsies (see 14 and 22 for classification scheme), 52 % had pulmonary microembolism (29), 60 % had pulmonary filling defects by occlusion angiography (22), while the majority had both macro- and microthrombi at autopsy (8, 22, 58, 74).

We found that coagulation laboratory screening tests (Table I) of patients who developed ARDS after thoracic and extrathora-

intravascular coagulation with fibrinolysis. Evaluation of the same plasma by specialized blood coagulation tests (Table II) showed that blood coagulation was activated in 60 % of the traumatized ARDS patients; laboratory screening tests of the same plasma led to a diagnosis of ICF in only 20 % (14 %).

Thus, a compensated state of intravascular coagulation with fibrinolysis appears quite common in post-traumatic ARDS patients.

1. Prothrombin time (> 13 sec)
2. Activated partial thromboplastin time (APTT) (>37 sec)
3. Fibrinogen level (<150mg%)
4. Platelet count (<150,000/mm$^3$)
5. Fibrin(ogen) degradation products (FDP's)(>20 μg/ml)

Table I. LABORATORY SCREENING TESTS FOR ICF. The criteria for positive ICF screen is 3 of the first 4 tests abnormal together with an elevated FDP level; abnormal values are in parentheses.

1. Increased soluble fibrin complexes (by plasma gel chromatography)
2. Increased fibrin(ogen) degradation products
3. Decreased factors V, VIII:C, and II
4. Decreased antithrombin III, $\alpha_2$-macroglobulin
5. Decreased plasminogen level

Table II. SPECIAL LABORATORY TEST FOR ICF. Criteria for diagnosis of ICF includes: increased amounts of SFC and FDP with 2 of the other 3 tests below the normal range.

a. What triggers blood activation in traumatized patients? The direct trigger of blood coagulation activation in traumatized patients appears to be the release of "tissue factor" at the site of injury. Tissue factor complexes with circulating blood coagulation factor VII, leading to thrombin generation and thrombus formation. This hypothesis has been challenged by Berman et al. (1969) (6) who postulated that platelets were activated at the site of tissue injury, that circulating platelet microaggregates subsequently lodged in the pulmonary circulation causing acute lung injury, and that activation of blood coagulation resulted from stimulation of platelets *in vivo* (6, 7). Although it is possible that platelet microaggregates are formed at the site of injury by the action of free arachidonic acid or thromboxane $A_2$ liberated from phospholipids, we believe that it is more likely that activation of platelets is a result rather than a cause of *in vivo* thrombin formation.

## 2. Intravascular coagulation without fibrinolysis

In a small subgroup of traumatized ARDS patients, intravascular coagulation is not associated with active fibrinolysis. Immediately post-trauma, an increase of circulating fatty acids liberated by the liver can have inhibitory effects on the tissue plasminogen of this subgroup of patients (61). This inadequate fibrinolysis, which we confirmed in 15 % of traumatized ARDS patients, may be secondary to genetic differences, obesity, hypertriglyceridemia, or other factors. One study reported that an increase of triglyceride-rich lipoprotein occurred in the plasma of post-traumatic patients with ARDS or fat embolism, but not in those who did not develop lung injury. This abnormal lipoprotein had an increased affinity for fibrin monomer. They postulated that lipoprotein-coated fibrin prevents plasmin from reaching its substrate or that it inhibits tissue plasminogen activator from generating plasmin. They showed that plasma levels of fibrin-rich triglycerids were positively correlated with the $(A\text{-}a)DO_2$ and were significantly higher in patients who died than in those who survived ARDS. In addition, the authors believe that fibrin-rich triglycerides provide a pathogenic mechanism for thromboembolism in post-traumatic ARDS patients (35).

The amount of fibrin deposited in pulmonary blood vessels depends upon the rate of fibrin formation and upon the mechanisms for fibrin dissolution and clearance by the lung. A competent fibrinolytic system and continuing pulmonary blood flow are essential to clear fibrin from the pulmonary circulation. If fibrin is modified by triglyceride-rich proteins, as suggested by Kunz et al. (1978)(35), its dissolution will be imparied, favoring pulmonary microthrombosis. Although it is unlikely that this abnormal lipoprotein is the sole cause of pulmonary thrombi in traumatized ARDS patients, it could potentially be an important factor accelerating pulmonary thrombosis.

## 3. In vivo detection of pulmonary fibrin deposition

### a. $^{125}$I-labelled human fibrinogen

Studies infusing $^{125}$I-labelled fibrinogen to detect fibrinogen deposition in the lungs of post-traumatic ARDS patients showed a shortened plasma fibrinogen survival time, an increased plasma fibrinogen turnover rate, and trapping of fibrin within the lung. Simultaneous measurements of blood coagulation factors and the degree of fibrinolysis did not discriminate between patients developing the microembolism syndrome and those who did not. Furthermore, fibrin trapping in the lungs, assessed by counting radioactivity over the chest, was reported at the onset of acute respiratory failure, suggesting a temporal relationship between fibrin thromboembolism and pulmonary injury (12). Although other investigators confirmed the findings of an enhanced fibrinogen turnover in post-traumatic ARDS patients and also, at autopsy, of pulmonary thromboembolism, they disagreed as to the accuracy of assessing $^{125}$I-fibrinogen radioactivity through the chest wall, which they felt underestimated the extent of pulmonary thrombosis found at autopsy (49).

### b. $^{99m}$Technetium (Tc-)-labelled human fibrinogen

Our group employed scanning of $^{99m}$Tc-labelled fibrinogen to localize areas of lung contusion in anesthetized dogs. We found that the contused areas were well-visualized by scanning the lungs if $^{99m}$Tc-fibrinogen was injected before contusion but not 15 mins. after the contusion. $^{99m}$Tc-fibrinogen radioactivity counts per gram of lung tissue were maximal at the center of the contusion and increased in the pericontused area as compared with normal lung tissue. $^{99m}$TC-fibrinogen activity remained high in the contusion site for at least 20 hours (20). With this canine model, we were able to demonstrate that this technique can easily detect an intrapulmonary "hematoma". In another model, intrapulmonary instillation of a 1 N HCL solution resulted in duffuse $^{99m}$Tc-labelled fibrinogen uptake by canine lungs.

More recently, our group extended the use of $^{99m}$Tc-labelled human fibrinogen to lung scanning of patients with ARDS. Fibrinogen uptake by the lung was determined by calculating the lung:heart radioactivity ratio at several times after injection. In a post-traumatic ARDS patient, areas of contusion in the lungs, heart, ribs, and femur were immediately visualized after $^{99m}$Tc-fibrinogen was intravenously injected. In patients with radiation pneumonitis or sepsis (Fig. 1), more diffuse pulmonary fibrinogen uptake was measured with a positive slope of the lung:heart radioactivity ratio. Patients recovering from severe ARDS continued to have a positive but fourfold decreased slope, while patients with mild ARDS exhibited a negative slope. In addition, localized areas of increased fibrinogen uptake were seen at sites of chest tube placement, rib fracture, arterial and venous puncture, suggesting that this technique is capable of visualizing localized thrombi, hemorrhage or edema, (53).

With this technique, scanning of the lungs and other organs is possible at the bedside with a high quality image. This represents an important advantage over the earlier $^{125}$I-labelled fibrinogen technique. However, unlike $^{125}$I-labelled fibrinogen, $^{99m}$TC-labelled fibrinogen lung scanning can only detect ongoing fibrin deposition or diffusion. Thus, we believe it will underestimate the extent of pulmonary thromboembolism found at autopsy.

Until more sensitive, specific techniques with high resolution can detect _in vivo_ pulmonary fibrin depositon, our understanding of the role of intravascular coagulation in lung injury patients will remain incomplete.

c. Can fibrin cause pulmonary injury?

The search to understand the effects of fibrin and its derivatives on the lung began in the mid-1960's. Bovine fibrinopeptide A and human fibrinopeptide A were given intravenously in minute concentrations to rabbits, dogs, and lambs and caused pulmonary hypertension, reduced lung compliance, and an increased (A-a) $DO_2$ (4). Saldeen's research group (1973) (57) was the first to postulate that pulmonary interstitial

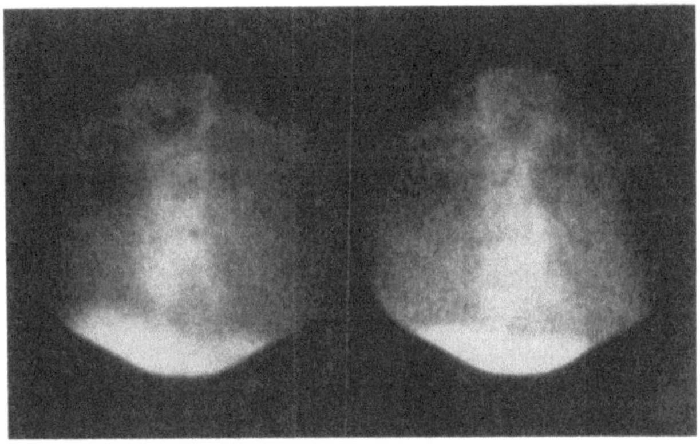

Figure 1

<u>$^{99m}$Tc-Human Fibrinogen Lung Scan of an ARF Patient.</u> The left and right scanning pictures were taken one and ten hours after $^{99m}$Tc-fibrinogen infusion, respectively. The patient suffered from Nocardia pneumonia and severe acute respiratory failure. Note a decreased uptake of $^{99m}$Tc-fibrinogen in the right upper lobe which corresponded to a large cavity.

and alveolar edema were the result of increased microvascular permeability caused by fibrin injury itself or by a derivative of fibrinolysis. They showed that only defibrinogenation had the protective effect of avoiding thrombin-induced pulmonary edema (11). In their studies, depletion of leukocytes, platelets, and complement or antihistamine therapy all failed to prevent thrombin-induced pulmonary edema. These observations were later confirmed by studies in which fibrinogen-depleted sheep failed to develop pulmonary vascular injury after thrombin injections (40). These investigators also confirmed that in the absence of fibrin, thrombin cannot induce pulmonary edema.

#### d. The relationship between fibrin deposition in the lung and increased pulmonary capillary permeability in ARDS

The "permeability factor" proposed by Saldeen's group (1973)

(7) has been identified as fibrin-peptide 6A. derived from the proteolysis of fibrin. This peptide inhibits antiotensin-converting enzyme (kinase II) which in turn potentiates the effects of bradykinin, a potent vasodilator (59). Thus, increased pulmonary capillary permeability associated with pulmonary fibrin deposition may not be caused by the direct effect of fibrin peptide 6A on the vessel wall, but by potentiation of the vasodilator effects of bradykinin.

Infusion of purified human fibrinogen fragment-D into awake rabbits causes progressive thrombocytopenia, depletion of complement, pulmonary dysfunction, increased pulmonary permeability to albumin, and neutrophil accumulation within the lung (44, 45). These authors previously measured increased Fg-D levels in the sera of ARDS patients and postulated that increased concentrations of circulating fibrin-D fragments may induce clinical acute lung injury (39, 45). If we assume that fibrin(ogen) fragment D, a product of plasma proteolysis of fibrin and fibrinogen, mediates pulmonary endothelial injury, we must also find another more direct trigger to activate the blood coagulation system. In traumatized ARDS patients this trigger may be the release of tissue factor at the site of injury. This would also explain the common finding of a prolonged prothrombin time and low plasma factor VII levels in traumatized-ARDS patients.

B. The hemostatic defect in non-traumatic ARDS

The two most common blood alterations reported in patients with acute respiratory failure secondary to aspiration, viral, or bacterial pneumonia, radiation pneumonitis, and septicemia are thrombocytopenia and increased circulating fibrin(ogen) degradation products.

1. Thrombocytopenia

a. Increased platelet destruction

Reduced platelet counts ($<100{,}000/mm^3$) were reported in 48 % of non-traumatic ARDS patients and hemorrhagic lungs in 33 % (28). The mortality rate (34 %) was twice as great in thrombocytopenic patients as in patients without thrombocytopenia (17 %). Disseminated intravascular coagulation was diagnosed in 50 % of the patients with thrombocytopenia. Among the remaining 50 % of patients with thrombocytopenia, 60 % had a prolonged prothrombin time and 30 % had increased levels of fibrin(ogen) degradation products (28). We suspect that patients who did not show evidence of ICF experienced a compensated state of intravascular coagulation which accounted for their increased platelet consumption.

Oppenheimer's group (1976) (52) reported thrombocytopenia in 93 % of patients with ARDS secondary to various bacterial infections (e.g., pneumonia), overt ICF in 35 %, and transient FDP elevations in 12 %. These authors suggested that although the blood screening tests (Table I) did not yield a diagnosis of ICF in the majority of patients compensated intravascular coagulation may have contributed to the reduction of circulating platelets. However, the authors also postulated other causes for thrombocytopenia, such as phagocytosis of bacteria by platelets, and bone marrow suppression by infectious agents.

Our group studied 15 patients with severe ARDS and found that thrombocytopenia was present in 50 % of these patients. Using $^{51}Cr$-labelled autologous platelets, we measured a shortened platelet survival (T 1/2 $2.3 \pm 0.39$ days, mean$\pm$SEM) compared with normal volunteers ($6.29 \pm 0.69$, $p<0.01$)(64). The platelet turnover rate in ARDS was twice the normal rate. Platelet sequestration, determined by surface scintillation counting, occurred rapidly in the liver, spleen, and to a more modest degree in the lungs.

Seventy percent of our thrombocytopenic patients had ICF diagnosed by blood screening tests and less than half had septicemia. Our results confirmed that the thrombocytopenia of the majority of ARDS patients appeared as a consequence of ICF. However, in a small group of patients, other factors may have been involved such as platelet phagocytosis of bacteria or viruses or platelets participating in thrombus formation. Although these studies did not determine whether platelets cause or exacerbate acute lung disease, the increased platelet consumption and pulmonary sequestration we detected suggested that platelets are directly involved in the pathophysiology of acute lung injury (64).

Recently, Spragg et al. (1982) (71) confirmed our results. Using $^{111}$In-labelled platelets in ARDS patients, they found a shortened platelet survival, as well as significant accumulation after three days of labelled platelets in the injured lung. Thus, platelets appear to participate locally in acute lung injury of diverse etiology. Whether activated platelets can induce pulmonary endothelial injury remains unknown. In septicemia and viremia, the platelet may be the primary agent inciting lung inflammation, rapidly joined by lung macrophages and leukocytes with subsequent fibrin formation and thrombosis.

b. Thrombocytopenia in ARDS may result from altered intrapulmonary platelet production

The provocative hypothesis that platelets are primarily produced by megakaryocyte fragmentation within the pulmonary circulation rather than by megakaryocyte budding in the bone marrow (46) is based upon substantial evidence accumulating since pulmonary megakaryocytes were first recognized (3). This observation has been repeatedly confirmed. The number of platelets in pulmonary venous blood is found to exceed that in pulmonary artery blood (30). In dogs with cardiopulmonary shunts, it has been demonstrated that the number of megakaryocytes in the lung is directly related to the flow of venous blood it receives (33).

Other investigators have observed the migration of whole megakaryocytes through bone sinusoidal endothelium by electron microscopy and question whether the pseudopodia and cytoplasmic protrusions previously considered to be platelets budding off megakaryocytes (75) instead were simply megakaryocytes entering bone marrow sinusoids (72).

The number and maturation of megakaryocytes in central venous and pulmonary artery blood differs from that in pulmonary venous and systemic arterial blood (32, 34, 62, 73). Usually, in central venous blood the megakaryocytes have been shown to have abundant cytoplasm as well as to be present in greater numbers than in the arterial circulation, where the cells are devoid of cytoplasm and markedly reduced in number. Taken together, the differences of platelet count and number, and the maturation of megakaryocytes prior to entering and after leaving the pulmonary circulation suggests that mature megakaryocytes give rise to platelets within the lung (18, 32).

The numbers of pulmonary megakaryocytes at autopsy have been shown to be increased in patients dying after trauma (10), thromboembolism (66, 68), intravascular coagulation, acute infections, cancer, blood loss, hapatic insufficiency, and shock (1). In the majority of these pathologic conditions, there is increased consumption of circulating platelets, and increased bone marrow megakaryocytopoiesis. Accordingly, the increase in pulmonary megakaryocytes found in these patients may reflect an increased number of circulating megakaryocytes. The large size of this cell's nucleus may increase their intrapulmonary trapping (46). Thus, these investigators propose that alterations of the pulmonary vasculature (e.g., in ARDS) or changes of megakaryocyte cytoplasmic volumes with concomitant alteration of structure produces platelets with a mean volume larger than the normal. Since large platelets are known to adhere and aggregate better than smaller platelets (42), they may accelerate thrombosis. In addition, several pulmonary pathological states may result from a dysfunction of pulmonary platelet production (46). Clearly, the thrombocytopenia we frequently measure in ARDS patients may result from both increased platelet destruction and "abnormal production". The latter required further clarification.

## 2. Fibrinolysis

### a. The nature and clinical significance of high levels of fibrinogen degradation products in the sera of ARDS patients

In 96 % if 80 non-traumatized ARDS patients, we found increased serum fibrin(ogen) degradation products (FDP). In the majority of these patients (76 %), we also found concomitant evidence of activation of the blood coagulation system with reduced concentrations of plasminogen, antiplasmins, and thrombocytopenia. The increase of FDP's in the sera of these patients was believed secondary to activated blood coagulation. In the remaining 20 % of ARDS patients, however, we found neither changes of plasminogen nor antiplasmins and believe that the elevated FDP levels in sera may have been produced by proteases other than plasmin. Furthermore, the only blood parameter that correlated with the increased FDP levels of these patients was an increased white cell count (over 10,000/$mm^3$). We postulate that leukocyte-elastase may have caused the proteolysis of fibrinogen we measured in these patients. Our results suggests that both plasmic and cellular fibrinolysis occur in ARDS patients. We do not know yet whether the peptide derivatives of plasmic and cellular fibrinolysis produce similar pathologic effects on pulmonary tissues.

Intravenous infusion in dogs of one plasmin-fibrinogen derivative, fragment D, has been shown to promptly induce acute lung injury (39, 43). Purified fibrinogen and its fragment D derivative have been demonstrated to stimulate the proliferation of hematopoietic cells *in vitro* (25) but their direct effect on cells in the vessel wall is unknown. Several workers have hypothesized that fibrinogen fragment D directly causes endothelial cell injury. This postulate has been strengthened by results measuring increased concentrations of fibrin(ogen) fragment D in the sera of patients with widespread endothelial damage, such as disseminated intravascular coagulation (5), thrombotic thrombocytopenic purpura (54), and ARDS (27, 55). Fibrin(ogen) fragment D has been found to be present in high concentrations in the blood of ARDS patients. The temporal relationship between fragment D and endothelial cell injury is uncertain; fibrin(ogen) fragment D elevation may not be the cause of endothelial cell injury in these pathological conditions but rather the result of it.

We shall now briefly review cellular fibrinolysis in ARDS.

### b. Cellular fibrinolysis in ARDS

In the bronchoalveolar lavage fluids (BAL) of ARDS patients, leukocyteelastase and other proteases are commonly found (37, 47, 48, 70). These proteolytic enzymes are uncommonly present in BAL of patients with other pulmonary diseases and are never detected in BAL of normal subjects (48). They conclude that leukocyte-elastase can contribute to lung injury during ARDS.

In isolated and perfused animal lung preparations, the intratracheal administration of leukocyte elastase caused protein-rich edema, but pulmonary tissue damage could not be histologically demonstrated (48) . This raises the question whether leukocyte elastase produces lung damage by itself or via the effects upon other mediators of inflammation, such as toxic fibrinogen derivatives.

c. Leukocyte elastase and blood coagulation changes during ARDS

Leukocyte-elastase *in vitro* rapidly activates fibrinogen, factors XII, VIII, and XIII, and has a moderate activating effect on factor V (63). In addition, *in vivo* infusions of leukocyte-elastase into Green monkeys resulted in a reduced plasma fibrinogen concentration, increased serum FDP level, and loss of factors II, V, VIII, and XII coagulant activities, but did not reduce the circulating platelet concentration (19). The proteolytic effects of leukocyte-elastase on blood coagulation proteins resemble those of plasmin but differ from the effects of thrombin since leukocyte-elastase spares platelets. It is therefore unlikely that intravascular coagulation in ARDS results solely from the effect of leukocyte elastase in blood. It is unknown whether elastase-fibrin(ogen) derivatives have an effect analogous to that of fragment D, a plasmin-fibrin(ogen) derivative, in increasing lung microvascular permeability.

d. Elastase-induced fibrinolysis by alveolar macrophages in ARDS

Like leukocytes, alveolar macrophages release elastase and other proteases that can activate complement and blood coagulation proteins. Endotoxin stimulation of leukocytes causes hydrolysis of fibrin by a white cell produced plasmin-type enzyme independent of plasma plasminogen activator. By a separate mechanism, endotoxin can induce macrophages to increase their membrane plasminogen activator and plasmin is immediately formed. In addition, endotoxin-stimulated macrophages secrete a proteinase that inhibits the activation of soluble plasminogen activator (15). Pulmonary macrophage-induced fibrinolysis may account for the elevated plasma FDP levels we measured in 20 % of ARDS patient without traumatic injuries in whom no other alterations of the fibrinolytic system were found.

The role of fibrinolysis in ARDS will not be understood until more is learned about the mechanisms of fibrinolysis. First, we must learn how to differentiate the fibrinogen derivatives produced by elastase from those produced by plasmin.

## CONTACT ACTIVATION OF BLOOD COAGULATION DURING ARDS

Intravascular coagulation with fibrinolysis is present in 60 % of patients with ARDS of various etiologies. To assess the role of Hageman factor activation in intravascular coagulation, we studied the plasma of 38 ARDS patients with septicemia and 24 ARDS patients with recent thoracic and extrathoracic trauma, all having similar degrees of lung dysfunction. We separated ARDS patients with chemical evidence of hepatic dysfunction from those without it. We measured the plasma levels of factor XII, prekallikrein, heavy molecular weight kininogen (HMWK), Cl inhibitor, and alpha$_2$-macroglobulin. Activation of the contact phase of blood coagulation was defined to have occurred if, at the same time, a) the levels of factors XII, prekallikrein, and kallikrein inhibitors were reduced and b) the functional prekallikrein level was found to be disproportionately low in comparison to the antigenic concentration of prekallikrein. Factor XII was significantly reduced in septic ARDS patients compared to patients developing ARDS after trauma ($p<0.01$). Both the functional and antigenic levels of prekallikrein were significantly reduced in patients with sepsis ($p<0.01$) but were not reduced in traumatized ARDS patients. There was disproportional reduction of functional prekallikrein in comparison with its antigen concentration in ARDS patients with septicemia. Thus, septic ARDS patients have an activated Hageman factor-kallikrein system, which can trigger intravascular coagulation and fibrinolysis. The intrinsic pathway of blood activation was not altered in patients suffering ARDS after traumatic injury. By examining which pathways of blood coagulation characterize these two major and differing etiologies of ARDS, this study provides insight into the relationship between blood coagulation changes and acute lung injury. If Hageman factor activation resulted solely from pulmonary endothelial injury, both groups of ARDS patients, with similar degrees of pulmonary damage, should have exhibit similar degrees of activation of the contact phase of blood coagulation. Since they did not, it is reasonable to postulate that in septicemia activation of the contact phase of blood coagulation may precede pulmonary injury while in post-traumatic ARDS this pathway of blood activation is not altered. Thus, it appears that the pathways of blood activation can vary with the etiology of ARDS. A more complete understanding of these mechanisms should lead to a rational therapeutic approach to the blood alterations of ARDS.

## ALTERED FACTOR VIII IN ARDS

Since pulmonary endothelial cell injury is universal in acute lung injury, factor VIII, a protein produced or released by endothelial cells and required for normal hemostasis, has been studied (13, 21). It has been postulated that disturbances of plasma factor VIII in ARDS might contribute to the deranged hemostasis of this syndrome.

Factor VIII circulates in the blood as a complex formed by two proteins with distinct biological activities in hemostasis: factor VIII coagulant (VIII:C), the cofactor required for rapid conversion of factor X to its activated form; and facor VIII von Willebrand's factor (VIII:vWF), which binds to a specific platelet receptor(s) and mediates the adhesion of platelets to subendothelial structures. (Figure 2). Factor VIII:vWF circulates in a multimeric form. Its larger multimers are essential for its biological action on platelets. This requirement appears to be due to the high affinity of this form of the VIII:vWF protein for platelet receptors as well as the ability of VIII:vWF to bridge the distance between platelets and induce their adhesion. The forms of VIII:vWF

# FACTOR VIII SYNTHESIS

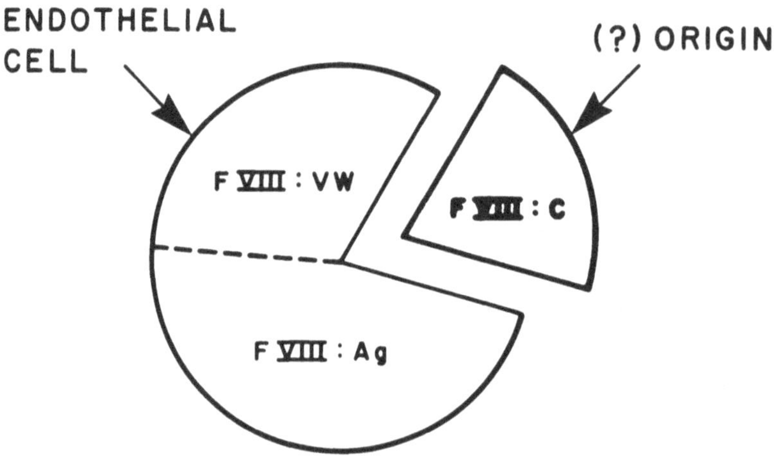


Figure 2

Factor VIII Synthesis. The non-shaded area represents the portion of factor VIII known to be synthesized by endothelial cells and measured by immunological techniques (VIII:Ag). This portion of the factor VIII molecule supports platelet adhesion and is called von Willebrand's factor (VIII:vWF); the shaded wedge represents factor VIII coagulant (VIII:C) activity (site of orgin unknown).

with a lower molecular weight exhibit this bridging ability only to a minimal extent. Selective deficiency of the larger VIII:vWF multimers results in a bleeding diathesis. Large multimeric VIII:vWF aggregates enhance the binding of a platelet membranes (56) and can increase platelet stickiness and promote thromboembolic complications.

In 12 women with overwhelming viral pneumonia, Grant et al. (1978)(21) reported factor VIII changes occurred during acute respiratory failure. They postulated that altered factor VIII might be a useful marker of pulmonary injury. They found that plasma factor VIII-related antigen (VIIIR:Ag) levels in these patients were markedly increased and out of proportion to the levels of factor VIII:C. Factor VIII:vWF activity was reported to be normal and correlated closely with VIII:C levels but not with VIII:Ag levels. All the ARDS patients had abnormal VIII:Ag patterns shown by crossed immunoelectrophoresis. These authors reported that factor VIII changes in ARDS correlated with the patients' clinical course.

We have confirmed and extended the factor VIII studies reported by Grant, Rodvien, and Mielke (1978) (21). In 100 ARDS patients, 29 critically ill patients without lung injury, and 60 normal subjects, we measured the plasma levels of VIII:Ag, VIII:C, and VIII.vWF. In addition, we studied the patterns of factor VIII electrophoretic mobility in 50 ARDS patients, 15 critically ill patients without lung injury, and 10 normal subjects.

On average, the plasma VIII:C activity in the ARDS patients was significantly elevated when compared to the normal subjects ($p<0.001$) or to patients without lung injury ($p<0.01$). There was a significant difference between VIII:C levels in patients without evidence of lung disease and normal subjects ($p<0.001$) (Fig. 3).

During ARDS plasma VIIIR:Ag increased up to fivefold the normal average ($p<0.001$) and twice the mean of patients without lung injury ($p<0.01$). Although the mean plasma VIIIR:Ag level of intensive care patients without lung injury was greater than normal, their increase was far smaller than that of acute lung injury patients (Fig. 4).

The mean VIII:vWF level for all 100 ARDS patients ($130 \pm 13\%$) was higher than normal ($p<0.01$); however, mean VIII:vWF decreased with increasing severity of lung injury. The highest levels of VIII:vWF ($204 \pm 14\%$) were measured in critically ill patients without lung injury and in patients with mild lung injury ($156 \pm 16\%$). These two groups differed significantly ($p<0.01$) from the normal subjects and from patients with severe lung injury (Fig. 5).

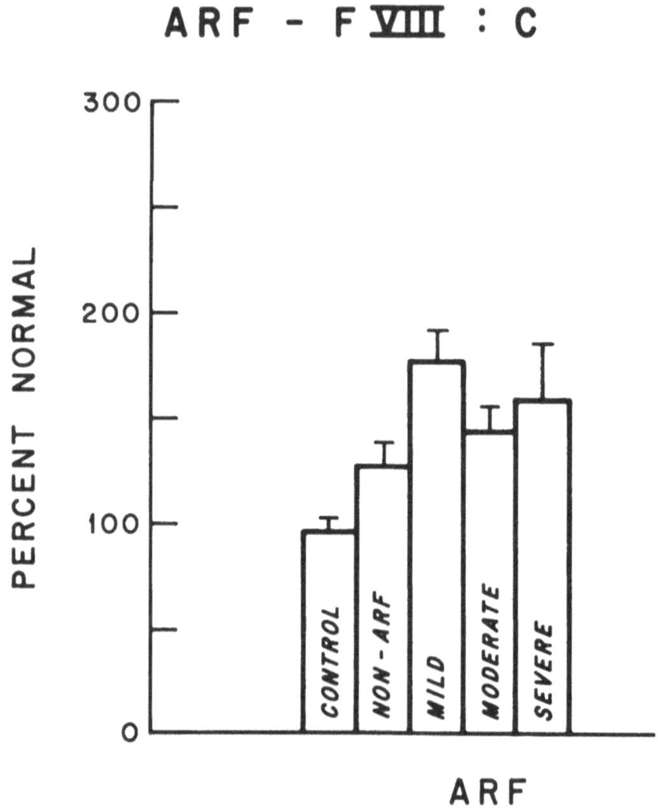


Figure 3

Factor VIII Coagulant Activity in Acute Respiratory Failure (ARF). The ordinate represents the factor VIII activity (VIII:C) as percent of normal pooled plasma (1 ml=100 %). The bars represent mean values and the vertical line one standard error of the mean. The bar labelled "non-ARF" represents the VIII:C results obtained in Intensive Care Unit patients without acute lung injury. The bars labelled mild, moderate, and severe show VIII:C values measured in ARF patients (see Carvalho et al, N. Engl. J. Med., 1982).

In ARDS patients, there was a remarkable disproportion between the levels of VIIIR:Ag and those of VIII:C and VIII:vWF. In the other critically ill patients without lung injury and in the normal group, these levels were in close proportion.

We demonstrated by crossed immunoelectrophoresis that in ARDS patients both the slowly and rapidly migrating factor VIII components had abnormal electrophoretic patterns; in moderate and severe ARDS patients their plasma contained a marked in-

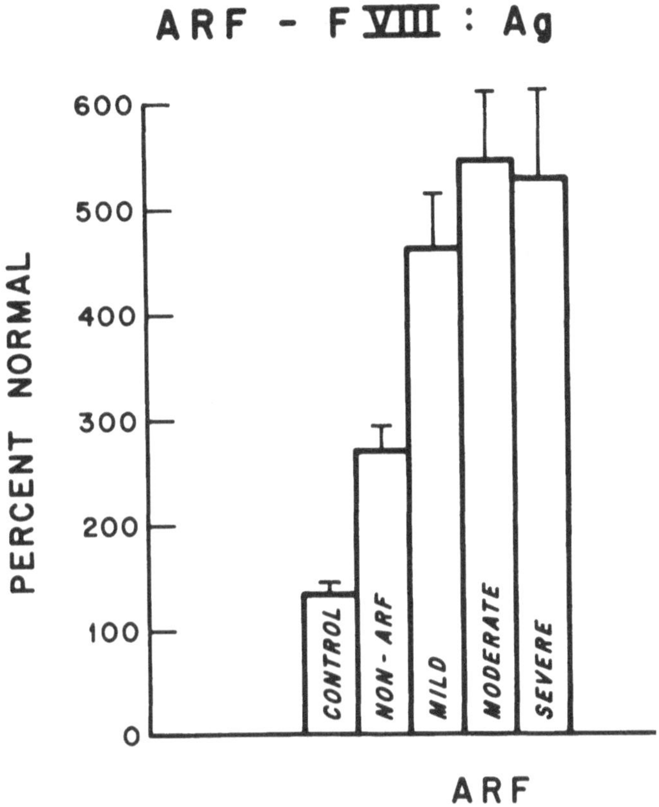


Figure 4

Factor VIII-Related Antigen (VIIIR:Ag) in ARF. The ordinate represents the VIIIR:Ag concentration expressed as percent of normal pooled plasma (1 ml = 100 %). The non-ARF bar represents the VIII:Ag levels of intensive care patients without ARF. The VIIIR:Ag concentration for ARF patients is represented by the bars labelled mild, moderate, and severe ARF.

crease of the factor VIII fast components (low molecular weight multimers) while in mild ARDS there were excessive amounts of slowly migrating factor VIII components (larger

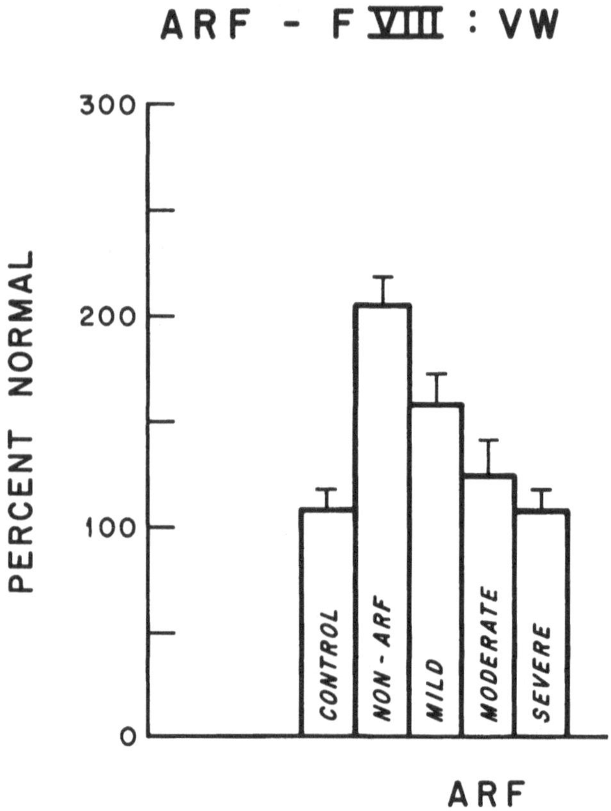


Figure 5

Factor VIII von Willebrand's Activity (VIII:vWF) in ARF. The ordinate represents VIII:vWF activity measured by ristocetin-induced aggregation of formalinized normal platelets suspended in the plasma of normal, non-ARF, and ARF patients. Each bar represents mean ± SEM.

molecular weight multimers). We postulated that the larger multimers of factor VIII present in excessive amounts in mild ARDS may increase platelet stickiness and promote pulmonary thromboembolism. In moderate and severe ARDS, patients with larger amounts of the smaller factor VIII components may have qcquired von Willebrand's disease and consequently a greater tendency to hemorrhage into the lung and elsewhere.

Patients who recovered from acute lung injury had factor VIII electrophoretic patterns that returned towards normal. Thus, VIIIR:Ag levels may provide ARDS-patients with a sensitive circulating indicator of pulmonary endothelial injury and repair.

## CONCLUSION

This review has presented a critical review of the known hemostatic defects of ARDS and their relationship to pulmonary endothelial injury. One of the most consistent blood changes found in patients with acute respiratory failure of diverse etiology is altered circulating factor VIII complexes. Since pulmonary endothelial injury is universal in acute lung injury and factor VIII is produced or released by endothelial cells, the excessive concentrations of factor VIII can be considered sensitive circulating indicators of pulmonary injury and repair. Because of the functions of factor VIII in hemostasis, altered factor VIII in ARDS may contribute to the thrombotic and hemorrhagic complications of ARDS.

Excessive fibrinolysis and thrombocytopenia are extremely common laboratory findings in ARDS patients. In the majority of cases, thrombocytopenia appears to be secondary to increased platelet consumption. However, the possibility of "pulmonary platelet sequestration" or "abnormal pulmonary platelet production" has been raised and must be further examined. The increase of serum fibrin(ogen) degradation products appears to be secondary to intravascular coagulation in most ARDS patients; however, a small subgroup of patients appears to exhibit cellular fibrinolysis without intravascular coagulation. Further studies are required to elucidate this point.

The etiologic factors of ARDS appear to dramatically influence the associated blood changes. Patients with septicemia most often had acute, decompensated intravascular coagulation with activation of the contact phase of blood coagulation, whereas patients suffering ARDS after trauma predominantly had compensated or overcompensated intravascular coagulation without evidence of contact activation of their blood.

Because both intravascular coagulation with fibrinolysis and acute lung injury share similar etiologic factors, the precise temporal and causal relationships between the two syndromes remains unclear. In general, it is believed that the hemostatic defects of ARDS are secondary to widespread primary pulmonary endothelial injury; however, there is growing experimental evidence to support an alternative pathway of lung damage induced by primary blood alterations. Thus, there are now various experimental animal models of ARDS that employ either activation of the blood coagulation system or activation of platelets or leukocytes to induce acute lung injury. Experimental data now exist to support possible toxic roles in the lung for fibrin, fibrin(ogen) fragment D, fibrin peptide 6A, elastase or its fibrin(ogen) derivatives, kallikrein, and other platelet (e.g., $TxA_2$, lipoxygenase derivatives) and leukocyte produced mediators (e.g., leukotrienes $LTC_4$, $LTD_4$) in the development of increased pulmonary capillary permeability and protein-rich pulmonary edema.

Finally, there is no doubt that during moderate and severe ARDS major and widespread deposition of fibrin in the lungs aggravates pulmonary function, leads to coagulative necrosis of the lung, and minimizes the chances for lung recovery (22).

We must continue to learn precisely how the coagulopathy of ARDS injures lung tissues. Early diagnosis and prompt therapy of intravascular coagulation may ameliorate the course of this devastating respiratory illness.

ACKNOWLEDGEMENTS

Supported by SCOR grant HL 23591.

REFERENCES

1. Aabo K, Hansen KB. Megakaryocytes in pulmonary blood vessels. 1. Incidence at autopsy, clinicopathological relations especially to disseminated intravascular coagulation. Acta Pathol Microbiol Scand Sect A 1978; 86: 285-291.

2. Anderson RR, Holliday RL, Driedger AA, Lefcoe M, Reid B, Sibbald WJ . Documentation of pulmonary capillary permeability in the adult respiratory distress syndrome accompanying human sepsis. Am Rev Respir Dis 1979; 119:869-877.

3. Aschoff L. Veber Capiliare Embolie Von Resenkerahaltigen Zellen. Arch Path Anat Phys 1893; 134:11-26.

4. Bayley T, Clements JA, Osbahr AJ. Pulmonary and circulatory effects of fibrinopeptides. Circ Res 1967; 21:469-485.

5. Bell WR. Disseminated intravascular coagulation. The Johns Hopkins Med J 1980; 146:289-299.

6. Berman IR, Gutierrez VS, Burrnan EL, Boatright RD. Intravascular microaggregation in young men with combat injuries. Surg Forum 1969; 20:14-16.

7. Berman IR, Smulson ME, Pattengale P, Schoenback SF. Pulmonary microembolism after soft tissue injury in primates. Surgery 1971; 70:246-253.

8. Blaisdell FW, Schlobohm RM. The respiratory distress syndrome: A review. Surgery 1973; 74:251-262.

9. Bone RC, Francis PB, Pierce AK. Intravascular coagulation associated with the adult respiratory distress syndrome. Am J Med 1976; 61:585-589.

10. Briu R, Halpren MM. The frequency of megakaryocytes in autopsy sections. Blood 1948; 3:286-291.

11. Busch C, Lindquist O, Saldeen T. Respiratory insufficiency in the dog induced by pulmonary microembolism and inhibition of fibrinolysis. Effect of defibrinogenation, leukopenia, and thrombocytopenia. Acta Chr Scand 1974; 140:255-266.

12. Busch C, Dahlgren S, Jakobson S, Jung B, Modig J, Saldeen T. The use of $^{125}$I-labelled fibrinogen for determination of fibrin trapping in the lungs of patients developing the microembolism syndrome. Acta Anesth Scand Suppl 1975; 57:46-54.

13. Carvalho ACA, Bellman SM, Saullo VJ, Zapol WM. Altered factor VIII in acute respiratory failure. N Engl J Med 1982; 307:1113-1119.

14. Carvalho AC, Saullo VJ, Bellman SM, Quinn D, Zapol VM. Intravascular coagulation in acute respiratory failure. Circulation 1982; 66(4):54.

15. Chapman HA Jr, Vavrin Z, Hibbs JB Jr. Macrophage fibrino-

lytic activity; identification of two pathways of plasmin formation by intact cells and of a plasminogen activator inhibitor. Cell 1982; 28:653-662.

16. Connors AF Jr, McCaffree DR, Rogers RM. The adult respiratory distress syndrome. In: Disease-a-Month 1981; Vol. 27. Chicago, Year Book Medical Publishers, Inc. pp 1-75.

17. Craddock PR, Fehr J, Brigham KL, Kronenberg RS, Jacob HS. Complement and leukocyte-mediated pulmonary dysfunction in hemodialysis. N Engl J Med 1977; 296:769-774.

18. Crosby WH. Normal platelet numbers. Pulmonary-platelet interactions. Ser Haemat 1976; 8:89-97.

19. Egbring R, Havemann K. Possible role of polymorphonuclear granulocyte proteases in blood coagulation. In Neutral Proteases of Human Polymorphonuclear Leukocytes. 1978; Edited by K. Havemann and R. Egbring. Baltimore-Munich, Urban and Schwarzenberg.

20. Geller E, Carvalho AC, Khaw B, Rajagopalan B, Strauss HW, Jones R, Zapol WM. Detection of canine lung contusion by $^{99m}$Tc-fibrinogen lung scan. J Trauma 1984; (In press).

21. Grant K, Rodvien R, Mielke CH Jr. Altered factor VIII complexes in patients with acute respiratory failure. Thromb Haemost 1978; 40:326-334.

22. Greene R, Zapol WM, Snider MT, Reid L, Snow R, O'Connell, RS, Novelline RA. Early bidside detection of pulmonary vascular occlusion during acute respiratory failure. Am Rev Respir Dis 1981; 124:593-601.

23. Hallman, M, Spragg R, Harrell JH, Moser KM, Gluck L. Evidence of lung surfactant obnormalities in respiratory failure. Study of bronchoalveolar lavage, phospholipid surface activity, phospholipase activiy, and plasma myoinositol. J Clin Invest 1982; 70:673-683.

24. Hammerschmidt DE, Weaver LJ, Hudson LD, Craddock PR, Jacob HS. Association of complement activation and elevatid plasma-C5a with adult repiratory distress syndrome. Lancet 1980; May 3, 1:947-949.

25. Hatfeld JA, Hatfeld A, Maigne J. Fibrinogen and its fragment D stimulate proliferation of duman hemopoietic cells in vitro. Proc Natl Acad Sci 1982; 79:6280-6284.

26. Hawiger J, Hawiger J Timmons S. Endotoxin-sensitive membrane component of human platelets. Nature 1975; 256: 125-127.

27. Haynes JB, Hyers TM, Giclas PC, Franks JJ, Petty TL. Elevated fibrinogen degradation products in adult respiratory distress syndrome. Am Rev Respir Dis 1980; 122: 841-847.

28. Hill RN, Shibel EM, Spragg RG, Moser KM. Adult respiratory distress syndrome; early predictors of mortality. Trans Am Soc Artif Intern Organs 1975; 21:199-204.

29. Hill JD, Ratcliff JL, Parrott JCW, Lamy M, Fallat RJ, Koeniger E, Yaeger EM, Whitmer G. Pulmonary pathology in acute respiratory insufficiency: lung biopsy as a diagnostic tool. J Thorac Cardiovasc Surg 1976; 71:64-72.

30. Howell WH, Donahue DP. The production of blood platelets in the lungs. J Exp Med 1939; 65:177-204.

31. Hudson LD, Adult respiratory distress syndrome. Seminar Respir Med 1981;2:99-174.

32. Kallinikos-Manikas A. Megakaryocytes and platelets in central venous and arterial blood. Acta Haematol 1969; 42:330-335.

33. Kaufman RM, Ziro R, Pollack S, Crosby WH. Circulating megakaryocytes and platelet release in the lungs. Blood 1965a; 26:720-721.

34. Kaufman RM, Ziro R, Pollack S, Crosby WH, Doberneck R. Origin of pulmonary megakaryocytes. Blood 1965b. 25: 767-775.

35. Kunz F, Hortnagl H, Kroesen G, Rumpl E. Plasma lipids, coagulation factors, and fibrin formation after severe multiple trauma in adult respiratory distress syndrome. J Trauma 1978; 18:115-120.

36. Lamy M, Fallat RJ, Koeniger E, Dietrich H-J, Ratlitt JL, Eberhart EC, Tucker HJ, Hill JD. Pathologic features and mechanisms of hypoxemia in adult respiratory distress syndrome. Am Rev Respir Dis 1976; 114:267-284.

37. Lee CT, Fein AM, Lippman M, Holtzman H, Kimbel P, Weinbaum G. Elastolytic activity in pulmonary lavage fluids from patients with adult respiratory distress syndrome. N Engl J Med 1981; 304:192-196.

38. Lung Program, National Heart and Lung Institute. Respiratory Diseases: Task Force on Problems, Research Approaches, Needs. Washington, D.C., Government Printing Office (DHEW publ. no. {NIH} 1972; 73-432, p. 171.

39. Luterman A, Manwaring D, Curreri PW. The role of fibrinogen degradation products in the pathogenesis of the respiratory distress syndrome. Surgery 1977; 82:703-709.

40. Malik AB, van der Zee H. Mechanisms of pulmonary edema induced by microembolization in dogs. Circ Res 1978; 42:72-79.

41. Malik AB, Lee BC, van der Zee H, Johnson A. The role of fibrin in the genesis of pulmonary edema after embolization in dogs. Circ Res 1979; 45:120-125.

42. Mannucci PM, Sharp MV. Platelet volume and shape in relation to aggregation and adhesion. Br J Haematol 1967; 13:604-617.

43. Manwaring D, Thorning D, Curreri PW. Mechanisms of acute pulmonary dysfunction induced by fibrinogen degradation products. Surgery 1978; 84:45-54.

44. Manwaring D, Curreri PW. The role of platelet aggregation and release in fragment D-induced pulmonary dysfunction. Ann Surg 1980; 192:103-107.

45. Manwaring D, Curreri PW. Platelet and neutrophil sequestration after fragment D-induced respiratory distress. Circ Shock 1982; 9:75-80.

46. Martin JF, Slater DN, Trowbridge EA. Abnormal intrapulmonary platelet production: a possible cause of vascular and lung disease. Lancet 1983; April 9:793-796.

47. McGuire WW, Cochrane CG, Spragg RG. Analysis of enzymes cleaving components of the Hageman factor (HF) system in the adult respiratory distress syndrome. Am Rev Respir Dis 1980; 121(Suppl.):275a.

48. McGuire WW, Spragg RG, Cohen AB, Cochrane CG. Studies on the pathogenesis of adult respiratory distress syndrome. J Clin Invest 1982; 69:543-553.

49. Mielke CH, Rodvien R, May N. Influence of extracorporeal membrane oxygenation (ECMO) upon the coagulation defect of acute respiratory insufficiency (ARI). Trans Am Soc Artif Intern Organs 1976; Abst 54.

50. Minna JD, Robboy SJ, Colman RW. Disseminated Intravascular Coagulation in Man. Springfield, IL, Charles C. Thomas Publishing 1974.

51. National Heart, Lung, and Blood Institute, Division of Lung Disease. Extracoporeal Support for Respiratory Insufficiency. Bethesda, MD, National Institutes of Health, pp. 243-245.

52. Oppenheimer L, Hyrniuk WM, Bishop AJ. Thrombocytopenia in severe bacterial infection. J Surg Res 1976; 20:211-214.

53. Quinn D, Geller E, Khaw B, Zielonka J, Barlaikovach M, Castorena G, Strauss HW, Carvalho AC, Zapol WM. Kinetics of $^{99m}$Tc-fibrinogen uptake by the lung in acute respiratory failure. Am Rev Respir Dis Suppl 1983; 127:87.

54. Ridolfi RL, Bell WR. Thrombotic thrombocytopenic purpura: Report of 25 cases and review of the literature. Medicine 1981; 60:413-428.

55. Rinaldo JE, Rogers RW. Adult Respiratory distress syndrome: Changing concepts of lung injury and repair. N Engl J Med 1982; 506:900-909.

56. Ruggeri ZM, Mannucci PM, Lombardi R, Federici AB, Zimmerman TS. Multimeric composition of factor VIII/von Willebrand's factor following administration of DDAVP: implications for pathophysiology and therapy of von Willebrand's disease subtypes. Blood 1982; 59:1272-1278.

57. Saldeen T, Busch C, Lindquist O. The effect of fibrin and platelets on the microembolism syndrome in the dog. Microvasc Res 1973; 6:256-258.

58. Saldeen T. Trends in microvascular research. The microembolism syndrome. Microvasc Res 1976; Microvasc Res 1976; 11:227-259.

59. Saldeen T, Ryan JW, Berryer P. A peptide derived from fibrin(ogen) inhibits antiotensin converting enzyme and potentiates the effects of bradykinin. Thromb Res 1981; 23:465-470.

60. Sanders AP, Baylin GJ. A common denominator in the etiology of ARDS. Med. Hypoth 1980; 6:951-965.

61. Sandler H, Diffang C, Gerdin B, Lindquist O, Saldeen T. The delayed microembolism syndrome: a review of 84 cases. Forens Sci 1976; 76:79-80.

62. Schein TM, Koivuniemi AP. Megakaryocytes in the pulmonary circulation. Blood 1962; 22:82-87.

63. Schmidt W, Egbring R, Havemann K. Effects of elastase-like and chymotrypsin-like proteases from human granulocytes on isolated clotting factors. Thromb Res 1974; 6: 315-324.

64. Schneider RC, Zapol WM, Carvalho AC. Platelet consumption and sequestration in severe acute respiratory failure. Am Rev Respir Dis 1980; 122:445-451.

65. Schumaker PR, Saba TM. Pulmonary gas exchange abnormalities following intravascular coagulation: reticuloendothelial involvement. Ann Surg 1980; 192:95-102.

66. Sharnoff JG. Increased pulmonary megakaryocytes-probable role in post-operative thromboembolism. JAMA 1959; 169: 688-691.

67. Shaw JO, Henson PM, Henson J, Webster RO. Lung inflammation induced by complement-derived chemotactic fragments in the alveolus. Lab Invest 1980; 42:547-558.

68. Smith EM, Butcher J. The incidence, distribution, and significance of megakaryocytes in normal and diseases human tissue. Blood 1952; 7:214-224.

69. Snow RL, Davies P, Pontoppidan H, Zapol WM, Reid L. Pulmonary vascular remodeling in ARDS. Am Rev Respir Dis 1982; 126:887-892.

70. Spragg RG, Cochrane CG and McGuire WW. Enzymatic activity causing cleavage of Hageman factor system components in human bronchoalveolar lavage fluid. Am Rev Respir Dis Suppl 1980; 121:279.

71. Spragg RG. Pulmonary platelet deposition. National Heart, Lung, and Blood Institute. Division of Lung Diseases. Excerpts from Pulmonary SCOR Progress Reports. Respiratory Failure 1982; 5:54-58.

72. Tavassoli M, Aoki M. Migration of entire megakaryocytes through the marrow blood barrier. Blood 1981; 48:25-29.

73. Tinggaard Pederson N. Occurrence of megakaryocytes in various vessels and their retention in the pulmonary capillaries in man. Scand J Haematol 1978; 21:369-375.

74. Tomashefski JF Jr, Davies P, Boggis C, Greene R, Zapol WM, Reid LM. The pulmonary vascular lesions of ARDS. Am J Pathol 1983; 112:112-126.

75. Wright JH. The histogenesis of the blood platelet. J Morphol 1910; 21:263-278.

# THROMBIN-INDUCED PULMONARY MICROEMBOLISM: MECHANISMS OF LUNG VASCULAR INJURY

ASRAR B MALIK, JOHN W FENTON II, ARNOLD JOHNSON, JEFFREY COOPER, RENA BIZIOS AND FRED L MINNEAR

Department of Physiology, Neil Hellman Medical Research Building, Albany Medical College of Union University, Albany, New York 12 208, USA

Division of Laboratories and Research, New York State Department of Health, Albany, New York 12 201, USA

and

Department of Biomedical Engineering, Rensselaer Polytechnic Institute, Troy, New York 12 181, USA

This review summarizes much of our recent data concerning the effects of thrombin-induced intravascular coagulation on the pulmonary microcirculation. We discuss the possible roles of several blood components (e.g. fibrinogen, platelets, and granulocytes) in mediating the pulmonary microcirculatory disturbances, and finally outline the pathways believed to be important in the development of lung vascular injury and pulmonary edema.

## 1. Effects of Thrombin on Pulmonary Microvasculature

### a. Morphological Alteration

Pulmonary morphological changes following thrombin-induced intravascular coagulation have been examined in a variety of species including the sheep, dog, and rat (15, 23). α-Thrombin, unlike other agents of inducing pulmonary microembolism, such as air, causes fibrin localization in the pulmonary vessels (Figure 1). The fibrin is present not only in pulmonary microvessels (i.e. vessels less than 50 μm in diameter) but also in larger (up to 300 um) vessels. This localization of fibrin in the lungs is a transient event which decreases within 3 hrs following thrombin injection (Table 1). The clearance of fibrin in this study in sheep lungs reflects the high fibrinolytic potential of pulmonary endothelial cells (19, 23).

Following thrombin-induced lung injury, platelets and neutrophils sequestration in pulmonary microvessels (Figure 2). Like fibrin, this is also time-dependent with neutrophil uptake occurring during the period 30 min to 3 hr after thrombin injection (Table 1). Neutrophils are found in close proximity to the fibrin deposits and are often in the process of degranulation (Figure 2). Platelet aggregation also occurs with evidence of degranulation (Figure 2). Therefore, α-thrombin induces not only intravascular coagulation by conversion of fibrinogen to fibrin but also pulmonary sequestration of neutrophils and platelets.

Interspecies differences must be noted in the thrombin-induced pulmonary microembolism model. No evidence has been obtained

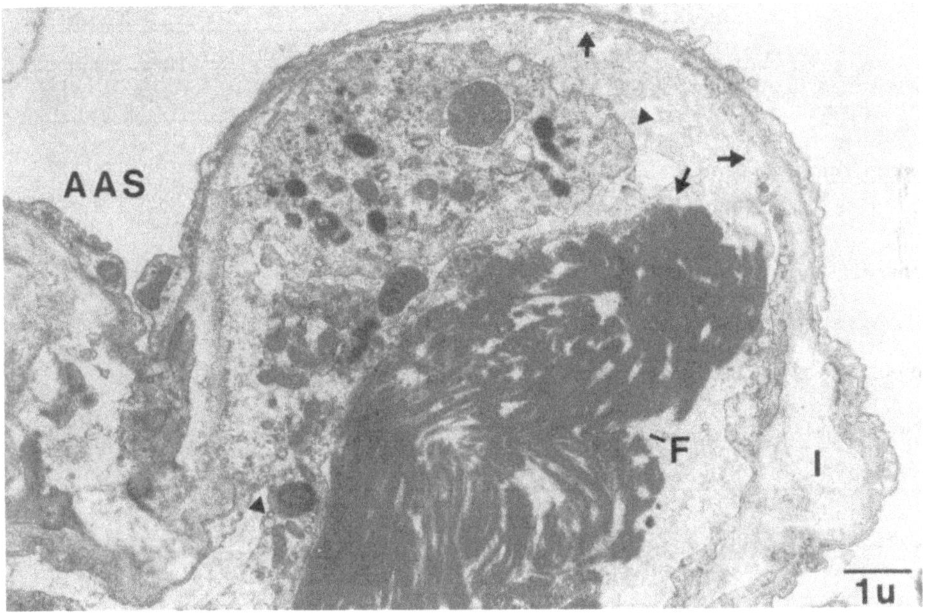


Figure 1

Electromicrograph of a dog lung 2-hrs after receiving α-thrombin. Intravascular fibrin is prominent and there are endothelial discontinuities indicative of endothelial injury (arrows). F=fibrin, I=interstitium, and AAS=alveolar space.

of interstitial fibrin accumulation in sheep lungs; however, interstitial fibrin has been observed in dogs and in patients with acute lung injury (17, 23), suggesting species differences in fibrinolytic activity. Although interstitial and alveolar edema was present as early as 30 min post α-thrombin injection, gross endothelial injury and denudation are not seen in the sheep lung (Figure 2). In dog lungs, interendothelial gap formations develop after thrombin, suggesting that this may be the pathway of increased transvascular fluid and protein exudation (Figure 1). In sheep, increased fluid and protein fluxes may result from increased endothelial-junction pore dimensions rather than gross endothelial injury (25, 28).

| | Leukocytes | | | Platelets | | | Fibrin Emboli | | |
|---|---|---|---|---|---|---|---|---|---|
| | min post infusion | | | min post infusion | | | min post infusion | | |
| | 0 | 30 | 180 | 0 | 30 | 180 | 0 | 30 | 180 |
| Experiment | | | | | | | | | |
| Sheep 1 | 38 | 69 | 53 | 19 | 77 | 5 | 0 | 54 | 3 |
| Sheep 2 | 26 | 24 | 61 | 23 | 15 | 17 | 0 | 9 | 13 |
| Sheep 3 | 57 | 35 | 107 | 14 | 10 | 41 | 0 | 45 | 21 |
| Sheep 4 | 27 | 46 | 41 | 47 | 15 | 18 | 2 | 11 | 2 |
| Sheep 5 | 53 | 42 | 76 | 65 | 33 | 34 | 0 | 29 | 2 |
| Means ± SEM | 40<br>±6 | 43<br>±7 | 68<br>±11 | 34<br>±34 | 30<br>±12 | 23<br>±6 | 0<br>0 | 30<br>±9 | 8<br>± 4 |

*Total number of leukocytes, platelets, and fibrin-deposits observed divi-did by total number of pulmonary vessels (< 20 μm in diameter) observed x 100.

TABLE 1. Morphometric Analysis of Leukocytes, Platelets, and Fibrin Sequestration in the Pulmonary Microvasculature. After Dose (44 μg/kg body weight) of α-Thrombin

b. Effects of Thrombin on Pulmonary Hemodynamics and Lung Fluid Balance

We have examined the pulmonary microcirculatory effects of thrombin-induced intravascular coagulation in the anesthetized dog and sheep (14, 16). Infusion of α-thrombin infusion results in large increases in pulmonary vascular permeability in both species (11, 16). An injection of α-thrombin (dosage of 100 clotting U/kg weight) in a typical sheep experiment resulted in a response shown in Figure 3. This dosage results in blood thrombin concentration of ~ 2 Units/ml, which occurs locally during activation of the coagulation cascade (5); therefore, this thrombin concentration would be expected to be present during intravascular coagulation. Thrombin resulted in transient but consistent increases in pulmonary arterial pressure and pulmonary vascular resistance (PVR) in this ani-

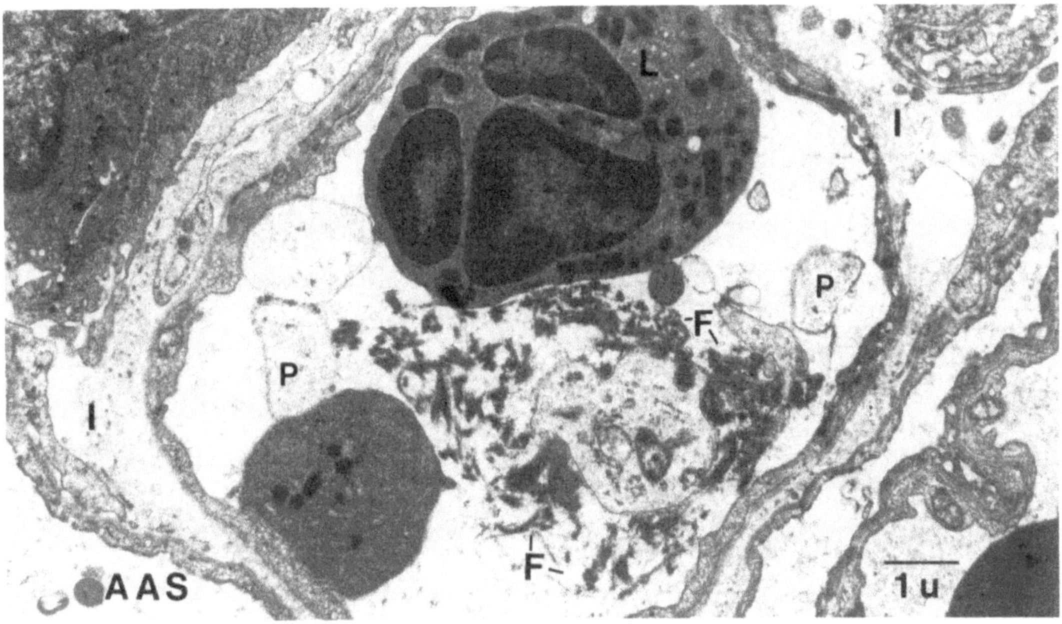


Figure 2

Electromicrograph of a sheep lung 30 min after receiving α-thrombin. Note leukocyte degranulated platelets (P), and intravascular fibrin (F). I=interstitium, AAS=alveolar space. Interstitial edema is also prominent at this time.

mal (Figure 3). More typically, both parameters remain elevated for up to 6 hrs, then gradually decrease towards baseline. These hemodynamic changes are associated with a marked increase in the pulmonary lymph flow (Qlym) reflecting an increase in the transcapillary rate of fluid filtration. In addition, the lymph-to-plasma total protein concentration (L/P) ratio is elevated, resulting in a marked increase in transvascular protein clearance ($\dot{Q}$lym x L/P ratio). This markedley increased clearance in the face of mildly elevated pulmonary vascular pressures and resistance indicates increased pulmonary vascular permeability.

A similar conclusion has been drawn in the dog model in which

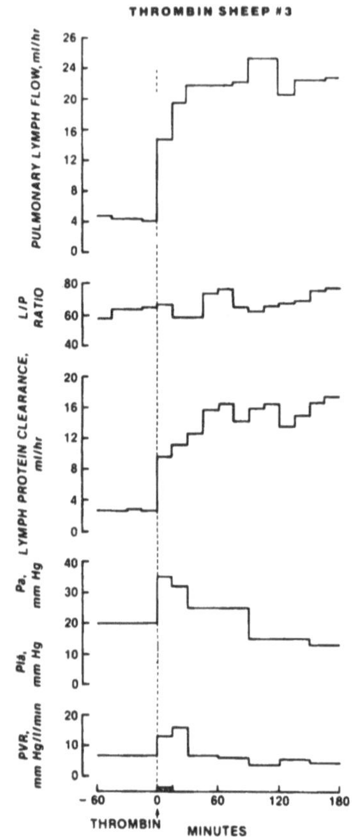


Figure 3

The time course of changes in pulmonary arterial pressure ($P_{pa}$), pulmonary vascular resistance (PVR), pulmonary lymph flow, lymph/plasma protein concentration ratio (L/P) and lymph protein clearance following α-thrombin in a typical sheep.

prenodal pulmonary lymph is collected and the protein reflection coefficient (σd) of pulmonary microvessels is determined (28). The normal σd in the dog lung is 0.72 (σd of 1 indicates that the microvascular barrier is impermeable to proteins, whereas σd of 0 indicates that it is freely permeable to proteins (28)). After thrombin-induced intravascular coagulation, σd decreased to 0.48 (16) demonstrating increased lung vascular permeability. Unlike other models of lung vascular injury, such as endotoxin (3) which does not increase lung vascular permeability in the dog lung (28), pulmonary microembolism increases permeability in both species.

Pulmonary edema is a characteristic lung response to microembolism (15, 23), and results from increased vascular permeability and microvascular pressure (23). Since the pulmonary arterial pressure is elevated after microembolization, the increase in the pressure may be transmitted to the injured pulmonary microvessels. An increase in hydrostatic pressure at a time when lung vascular permeability is increased will greatly enhance the fluid filtration rate. Therefore, for a given increase in microvascular pressure, the fluid filtration rate in thrombin-embolized lungs is greater than in the normal lung (15).

d. Dosage Response

The pulmonary-lymph response is dependent on the dosage of α-thrombin (Figure 4). This incremental response most likely results from dose-independent increases in lung vascular permeability since it is not associated with dose-dependent increases in pulmonary arterial pressure and PVR. The importance of this finding is that the increase in lung vascular permeability can be graded. If the mechanism of the increased permeability is being examined, this necessitates the assessment of permeability at similar thrombin dosages.

d. Response in Unanesthetized Animals

Differences exist in the pulmonary vascular response to thrombininduced intravascular coagulation between halothane-anesthetized acutely prepared sheep and chronically-instrumented awake animals. The same dosage of α-thrombin (100 U/kg body weight) which induces sustained increases in pulmonary arterial pressure and PVR in the anesthetized-acutely prepared animal does not result in sustained responses in the awake animal. This is consistent with observations that surgical trauma and anesthesia inhibit fibrinolysis (23). Pretreatment of awake sheep with tranexamic acid (to partially inhibit fibrinolysis), however, caused sustained increases in pulmonary arterial pressure and PVR after thrombin. In addition, pulmonary lymph flow and transvascular protein clearance increased markedly and were maintained for up to 10 hrs (Figure 5). These findings suggest that fibrinolytic activity modulates the pulmonary vascular permeability response to intravascular coagulation. The clot retention time in the pulmonary microcirculation (which is determined by the fibri-

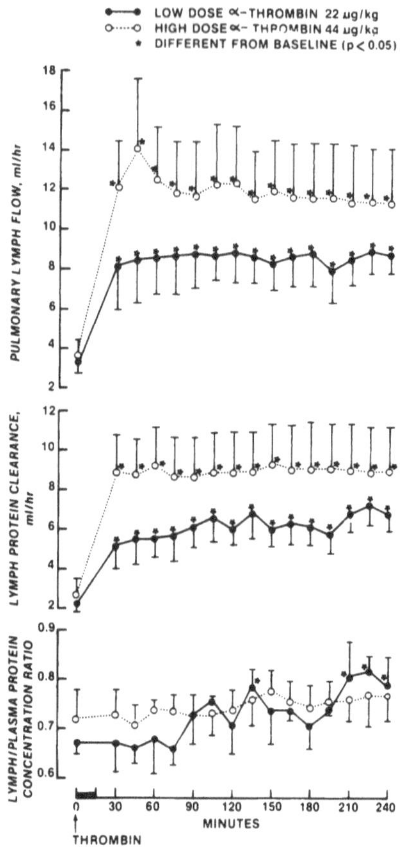


Figure 4

Pulmonary lymph flow, lymph/plasma protein concentration ratio, and lymph protein clearance and after α-thrombin in the low dose (22 ug/kg) and high dose (44 ug/kg) α-thrombin groups.

nolytic activity) may be an important determinant of lung vascular injury.

e. Intravascular Coagulation Development of Lung Vascular Injury.

Alpha-thrombin has a high fibrinogen clotting activity as well as other functions, such as platelet aggregation and leukocyte chemotaxis (5). In contrast, γ-thrombin, which is formed *in vivo* by autoproteolysis or *in vitro* by limited trypsin digestion of α-thrombin (5), lacks clotting activity yet retains certain other thrombin-ascribed activities (Table II and III). Both thrombins maintain their ability to cleave synthetic substrates and are inactivated by anti-thrombin III (5). However, platelet activation and aggregation is an order

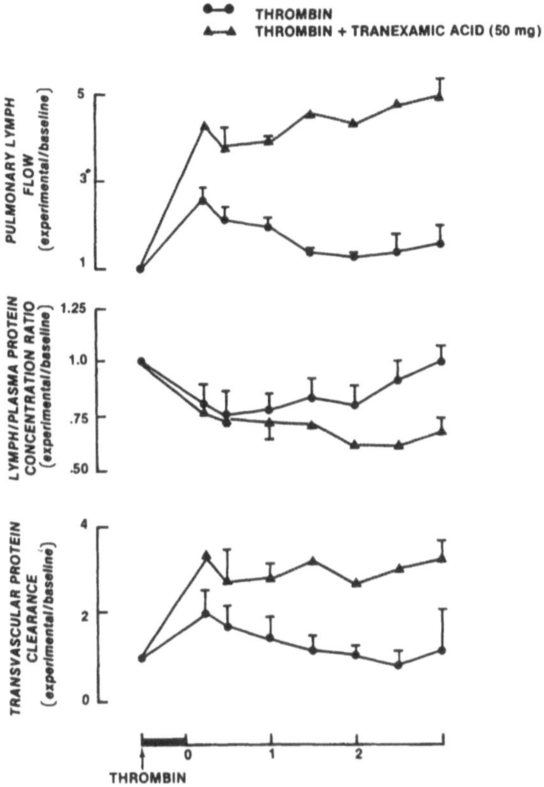


Figure 5

The time course of changes in pulmonary lymph flow, lymph/plasma protein concentration ratio, and transvascular protein clearance following α-thrombin in awake sheep. A small amount of tranexamic acid was injected in one group to prolong clot retention in the awake animal.

of magnitude less and fibrinogen clotting activity is negligible for γ-thrombin (15). This marked loss of fibrinogen clotting is attributable to a destruction of the fibrinogen recognition site on the "fibrinside" of catalytic site of α-thrombin (5).

The functional differences of α- and γ-thrombin are reflected in their relative abilities to change the blood concentrations of platelets, leukocytes, and fibrinogen _in vivo._ The decrease in platelet count after injection of α-thrombin was marked and sustained in contrast to the small and relatively transient decrease after γ-thrombin. This was also the case with the changes in the leukocyte count. Fibrinogen concentration decreased immediately after injection of α-thrombin,

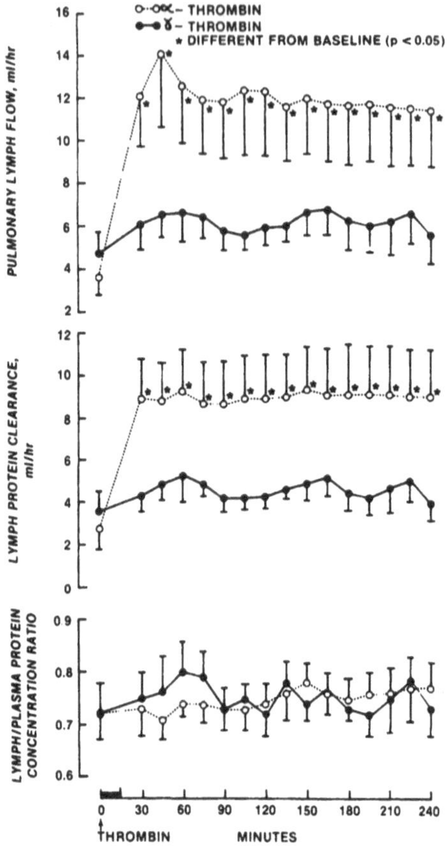


Figure 6

Pulmonary lymph flow, lymph/plasma protein concentration ratio, and lymph protein clearance after infusion of α-thrombin and γ-thrombin

while a minimal change occurred after γ-thrombin (Figure 6). The lack of fibrinogen consumption is also reflected in the finding that the concentration of fibrin degradation products did not increase after α-thrombin.

Infusion of γ-thrombin at a molar dosage equivalent to α-thrombin is not followed by increases in pulmonary lymph flow and transvascular protein clearance (Figure 6). This response is in sharp contrast to that observed after α-thrombin (Figure 6), indicating that intravascular coagulation and fibrinolytic activation are required for increased lung vascular permeability. This does not preclude the possibility, that lung vascular injury after microembolism can

| Property | α-Thrombin | γ-Thrombin |
|---|---|---|
| Molecular Weight | ~36,600 | ~36,600 |
| Chain Structure | 2 covalent chains | 3 Noncovalent Chains β-chain fragment; each contribute to the active site |
| Enzymatic Activities | High fibrinogen-clotting and all other thrombin-ascribed activities | Equivalent synthetic substrate activities and reacticity with antithrombin III and $\alpha_2$-macroglobulin; reduced platelet stimulatory and monocyte activities |
| Physiologic Importance | Central bioregulatory enzyme in hemostasis; product of thromboplastin activation of prothrombin | Unknown; could be formed in pancreas, where trypsin activates prothrombin |

TABLE II. Properties of Human α- and γ-Thrombin

| Activity | α/γ-ratio |
|---|---|
| Synthetic substrate cleavage | ~1 |
| Antithrombin III inactivation | ~1 |
| Factor XIII activation | <10 |
| Platelet stimulatory | ~10 |
| Fibrinogen clotting | ~3,000 |

TABLE III. Relative Activities of α- and γ-Thrombins

occur independently of intravascular coagulation, as is the case after air embolism in which there is no intravascular coagulation (7, 20). Therefore, intravascular coagulation most probably initiates thrombin-induced lung vascular injury, but is not the final effector of the injury.

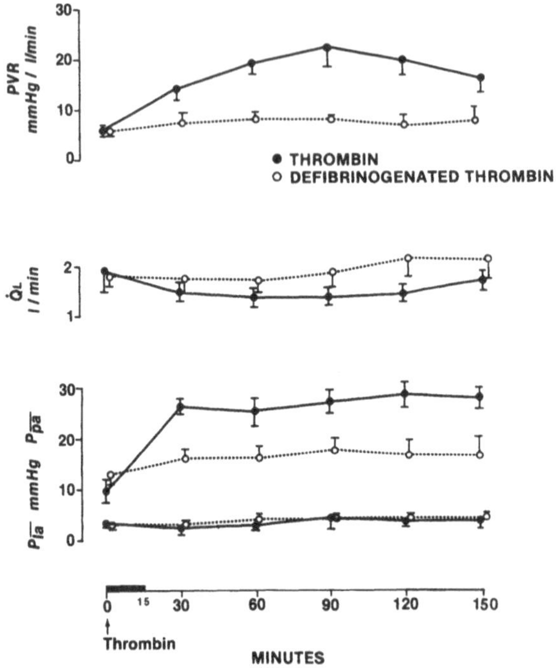


Figure 7

Pulmonary vascular resistence (PVR), pulmonary blood flow ($Q_L$), mean pulmonary arterial pressure ($P_{\overline{pa}}$), and mean left atrial pressure ($P_{\overline{la}}$) following α- thrombin in control and defibrinogenated groups.

## 2. Role of Blood Components

Since accumulations of fibrin, leukocytes, and platelets in pulmonary microvessels are prominent features of thrombin-induced intravascular coagulation, we have examined interactions among these blood components in mediating lung vascular injury.

### a. Fibrin

The contribution of fibrinogen was examined in fibrinogen depletion studies. Fibrinogen was depleted in intact sheep using a purified fraction of Malayan pit viper venom (Ancrod) (1, 10). Chronic administration of the fraction resulted in plasma fibrinogen concentrations approaching zero. Administration of α-thrombin in these animals decreased the platelet

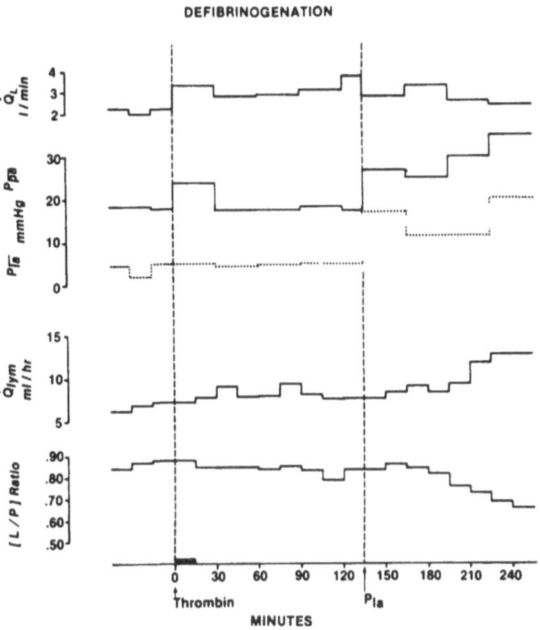


Figure 8

Pulmonary lymph flow (Qlym), lymph/plasma protein concentration ratio (L/P), pulmonary blood flow ($Q_L$); mean pulmonary arterial pressure ($P_{\overline{pa}}$) and mean left atrial pressure ($P_{\overline{la}}$) following α-thrombin in a defibrinogena.

counts comparable to those observed in the control group receiving the same amount of thrombin, indicating an effective platelet aggregation in either group. However, the leukocyte count does not decrease and pulmonary arterial pressure and PVR do not increase as in the control group (Figure 7). Therefore, pulmonary hypertension and increased PVR after thrombin infusion are related to intravascular coagulation. Intravascular coagulation may induce these hemodynamic changes by obstruction of pulmonary vessels, as well as by release of vasoactive humoral mediators (15, 22, 23).

Defibrinogenation also prevented to a large extent the thrombin-induced increases in pulmonary lymph flow and transvascular protein clearance (Figure 8). Moreover, raising the pulmonary capillary pressure by inflation of left atrial balloon, resulted in an increase in pulmonary lymph flow and a decrease in lymph-to-plasma protein concentration ratio indicating that the sieving properties of the pulmonary microvasculature were not altered. In the control-thrombin group, the increase in pulmonary lymph flow after induction of capillary hypertension was associated with an no changes in lymph-to-plasma protein concentration ratio. Saldeen (23) observed that fibrinogen is required for the expression of pulmonary edema after thrombin challenge, and we have amplified these observations by showing that thrombin mediates the increase in lung vascular permeability by converting fib-

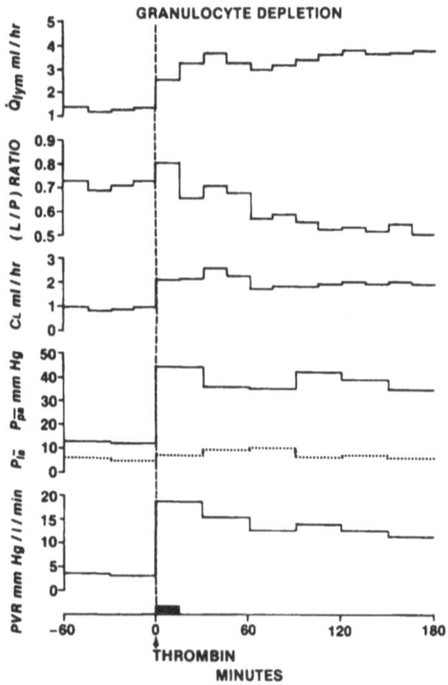


Figure 9

Pulmonary lymph flow (Qlym), lymph/plasma protein concentration ratio (L/P), lymph protein clearance ($C_L$), mean pulmonary arterial pressure ($P\overline{pa}$), left atrial pressure ($P\overline{la}$), and pulmonary vascular resistance (PVR), following α-thrombin in a sheep made granulocytopenic with hydroxyurea

rinogen to fibrin and that subsequent fibrinolysis is required for the overall process.

b. Leukocytes

The infusion of α-thrombin into an animal selectively granulocytedepleted with hydroxyurea (cell count 200 cells/ml) increases pulmonary lymph flow but to a lesser extent than in the control group (Figure 9). This increase is associated with the decrease in lymph-to-plasma protein concentration ratio, indicating an increased movement of water. This could be the result of an increase in capillary pressure occurring as a result of thrombin-induced embolism; but, it cannot be explained by an increase in lung vascular permeability because this would have resulted in an unchanged or even a higher lymph-to-plasma protein ratio during the increased pulmonary lymph flow (23). The permeability increase response to thrombin is also prevented by neutrophil depletion-induced antineutrophil serum (Figure 9a).

Therefore, granulocytes are the key effectors of the increased lung vascular permeability after microembolism. Granulocytes are also responsible for the increase in extravascular lung water which occurs after microembolism (27).

Morphometric data show that leukocytes are attracted to the pulmonary circulation following thrombin-induced intravascular coagulation (Table I). Consistent with the morphometric data (Table I), thrombin injection results in an increase in activity in the lung as measured by gamma scintigraphy of $^{111}$Indium-oxine labelled sheep leukocytes (Figure 10). Leukocytes appear to mediate the lung injury and then leave the pulmonary circulation. Pulmonary microembolism-induced injury is an acute event resulting from a transiet migration and uptake of neutrophils following thrombin-induced intravascular coagulation.

c. Platelets

Unlike the effect of granulocyte depletion in preventing the increase in lung vascular permeability, depletion of platelets (a circulating count <10,000 cells/ul) does not inhibit the

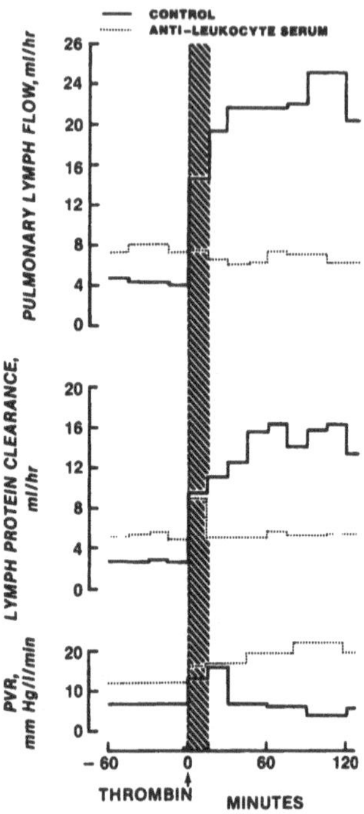


Figure 9a

Pulmonary hemodynamic and lymph responses after α-thrombin in a sheep made granulocytopenic with anti-leukocyte serum

permeability-increase. Injection of thrombin into platelet-depleted animals results in an increased pulmonary lymph flow (although much smaller than in the control group) and in an increase in lymph-to-plasma protein concentration ratio (Figure 11). Moreover, raising the pulmonary capillary pressure, by inflating a left atrial balloon, produces a relatively large increase in lymph flow not associated with a decrease in lymph-to-plasma protein ratio, indicating increased protein sieving as in the control-thrombin group (Figure 11a).

Although platelet depletion clearly did not prevent the per-meability increase, it produced much smaller increases in pul-

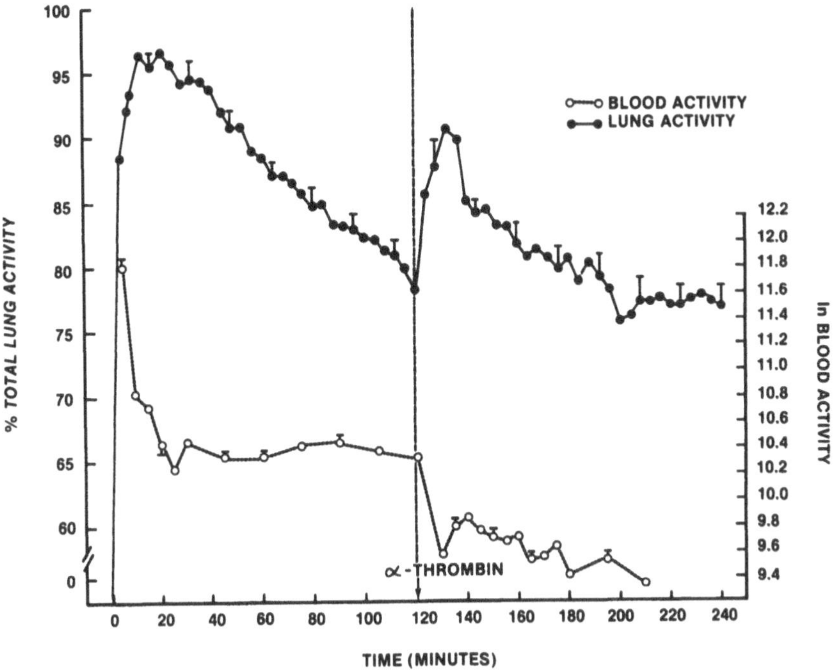


Figure 10

$^{111}$Indium activity of the lung and blood following injection of $^{111}$Indium-labelled leukocytes. α-thrombin was injected at 120 min.

monary fluid filtration after thrombin-induced intravascular coagulation. The reason for this response is not clear; one possible mechanism is that in the absence of circulating platelets there is no subsequent platelet aggregation and/or release of vasoconstrictor mediators, such as thromboxane $A_2$ and serotonin (29). Therefore, platelet aggregation probably contributes to pulmonary edema by raising capillary pressure, but it does not contribute to the increase in lung vascular permeability.

d. Oxygen Radicals

Generations of oxygen radicals secondary to leukocyte activation (29) may be important in the mediation of lung vascular injury after α-thrombin. Leukocyte activation causes the generation of toxic oxygen metabolites, such as the superoxide

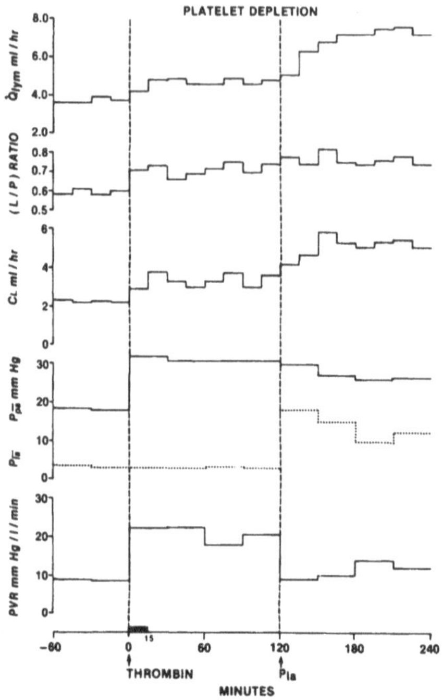


Figure 11

Pulmonary lymph flow (Qlym), lymph/plasma protein concentration ratio (L/P), transvascular protein clearance ($C_L$), mean pulmonary arterial pressure ($P_{\overline{pa}}$), mean left atrial pressure ($P_{\overline{la}}$), and pulmonary vascular resistance (PVR) after α-thrombin in thrombocytopenic sheep.

anion, hydrogen peroxide, and hydroxyl radical (4, 21). Superoxide dismutase catalyzes the conversion of superoxide anions to hydrogen peroxide and oxygen. Superoxide dismutase bound to Ficoll has a prolonged circulating life and is distributed in the interstitium following intravenous injection (21). In animals pretreated with superoxide dismutase-Ficoll, the increase in lymph flow after thrombin is blunted but not completely inhibited (Fig. 9b). Similar results are observed with air embolism (6). Therefore, the generation of superoxide anions is important in the development of increased lung vascular permeability after thrombin-induced intravascular coagulation.

The most vasotoxic oxygen radical cannot be assessed from this type of study. Hydroxyl radicals could be as important as superoxide anions since formation of hydroxyl radicals by the

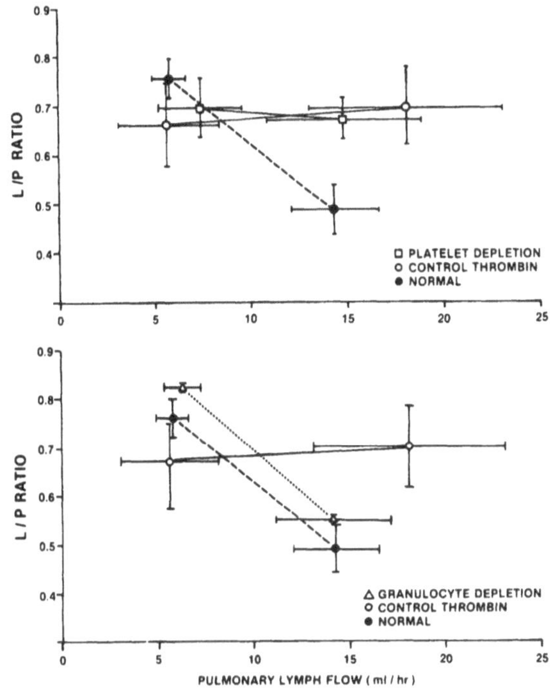


Figure 11a

Pulmonary lymph flow versus the lymph/plasma protein concentration ratio (L/P) after left atrial hypertension in normal, control-thrombin, and platelet-depleted thrombin groups (above). Note the different response after thrombin in the granulocyte-depleted group (below)

Haber-Weiss reaction requires both $H_2O_2$ and superoxide anion. Thus, the overall protective effect of superoxide dismutase may be due to removal of superoxide anions and to the subsequent lack of formation of hyroxyl radicals.

### 3. Mediation of Leukocyte-Dependent Lung Vascular Injury After Thrombin

Little is known about the mechanisms of leukocyte activation after intravascular coagulation and how these are involved in the development of lung vascular injury. The following section discusses the potential pathways of leukocyte activation.

#### a. Plasminogen Activation

Inhibition of plasminogen activation can be examined by using

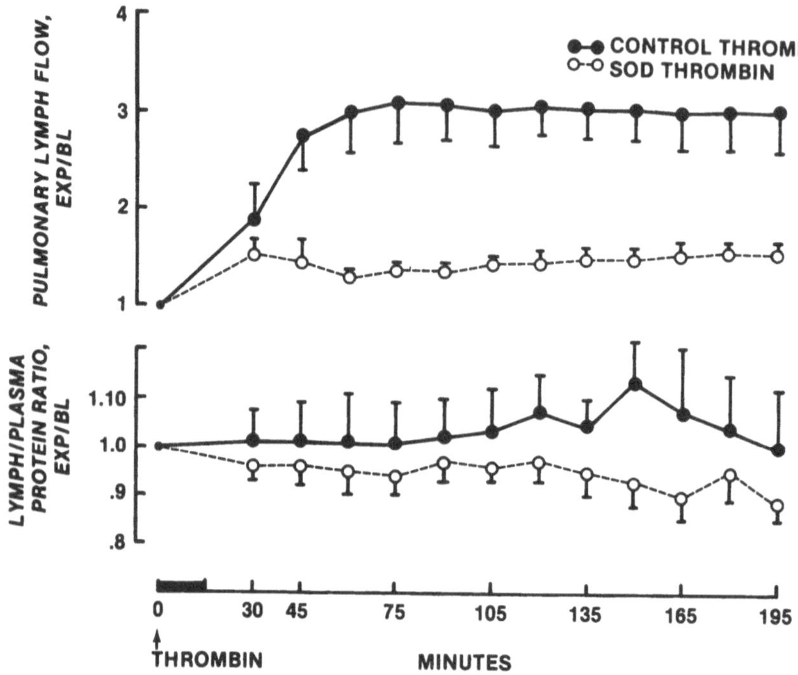


Figure 9b

Pulmonary lymph flow and lymph-plasma protein concentration ratio after α-thrombin in control and superoxide dismutase-pretreated groups

tranexamic acid, a compound which binds to tissue plasminogen activator and prevents the conversation of plasminogen to plasmin (19). Following α-thrombin infusion in the tranexamic acid-treated group, the concentration of fibrin degradation products does not increase despite the fibrinogen consumption (Figure 12), indicating complete inhibition of fibrinolytic activity. Platelet count decreases comparably in both groups while the leukocyte count in the tranexamic acid group did not decrease as in the control group. A delayed increase in pulmonary lymph flow after α-thrombin is associated with a decrease in the lymph-to-plasma protein concentration ratio (Figure 13). Raising left atrial pressure in these animals

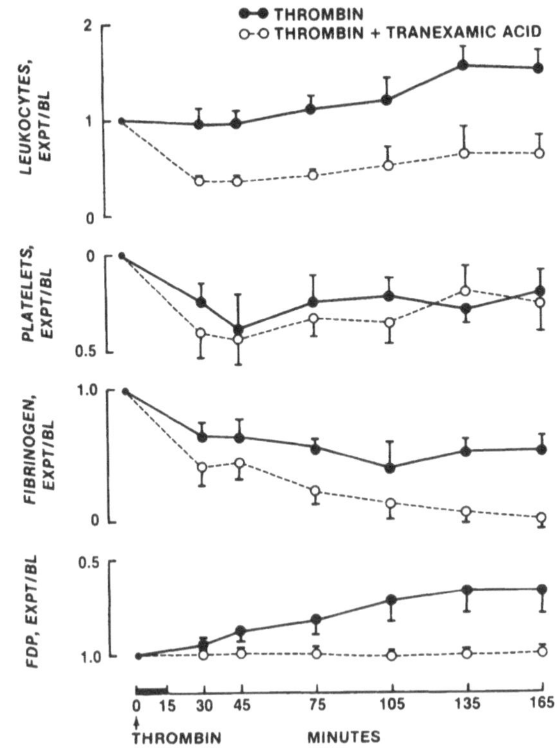


Figure 12

Leukocyte, platelet, fibrinogen, and fibrin degradation product (FDP) levels after α-thrombin in the control-thrombin and fibrinolysis-inhibited groups (tranexaminc acid-treated)

results in increased lymph flow and a further decrease in lymph-to-plasma protein concentration ratio comparable to the effects of capillary hypertension in the normal group. Therefore, fibrinolysis is necessary for the increase in lung vascular permeability, perhaps through formation of fibrin degradation products (23) and subsequent activation of plasminogen-dependent pathways (11, 12, 23).

Fibrinolytic inhibition prevents both the uptake of $^{111}$Indium oxinelabelled neutrophils in the lungs and the concomitant decrease in peripheral leukocyte count after administration of α-thrombin (Figure 14). Plasminogen activation thus appears to be required for the mediation of leukocyte sequestration in the lung. We propose that the prevention of pulmonary injury by fibrinolytic inhibition is due to the inhibition of

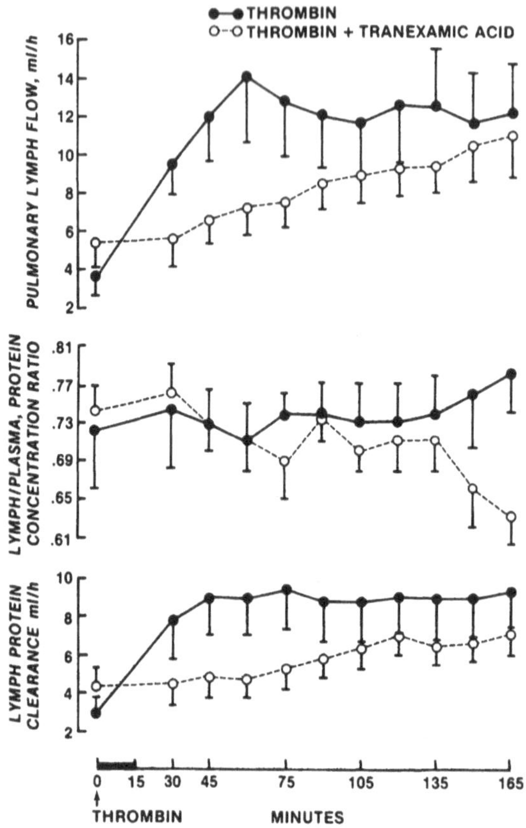


Figure 13

Pulmonary lymph flow, lymph/plasma protein concentration ratio and lymph protein clearance after α-thrombin in the control thrombin and fibrinolysis inhibited (tranexamic acid-treated) thrombin groups.

leukocyte uptake in the lung.

b. Complement Activation

The generation of plasmin results in cleavage of complement protein and generation of complement-derived chemotactic peptides (18, 22, 26). When total hemolytic complement activity is reduced to below 30 % of baseline using purified cobra venom factor (9, 18), thrombin infusion results in a transient increase in pulmonary lymph flow compared to that observed in the control group (Fig. 15). Another major difference is a decrease in the lymph-to-plasma protein ratio (Figure 15). This response is remarkably similar to that observed in the granulocyte-depleted animals (Figure 9). In the complement-depleted animals, marked or sustained in-

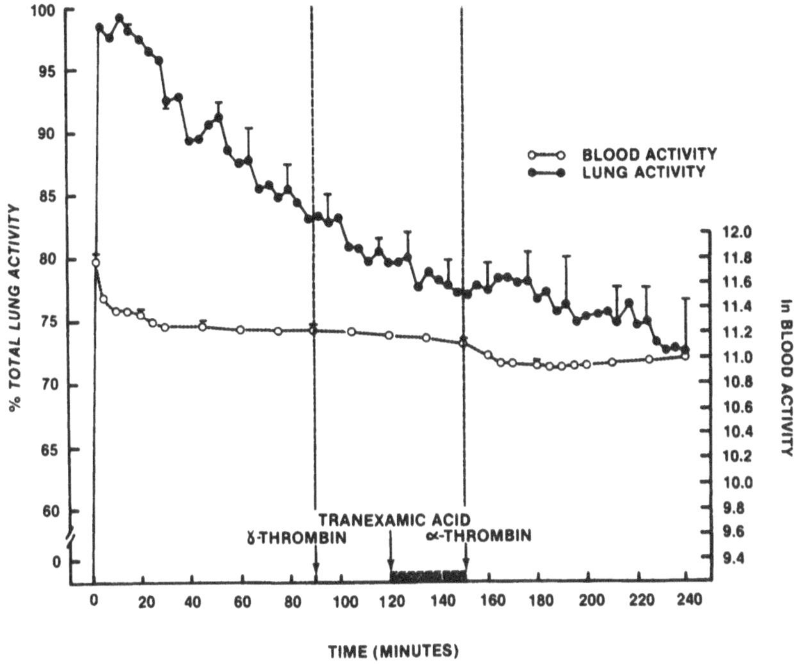


Figure 14

[111]Indium activity of the lung and blood following injection of [111]Indium-labelled leukocytes. Note that γ-thrombin (unlike α-thrombin in Figure 10) had no effect on neutrophil uptake. Also, fibrinolysis-inhibition with tranexamic acid largeley prevented the neutrophil uptake after injection of α-thrombin at 150 min.

increases in the leukocyte count do not occur. The effect of complement depletion in preventing the increase in lung vascular permeability may be due to the absence of complement-derived peptides (C3a and C5a), which have leukocyte aggregating and activating properties (18, 29).

The basis for leukocyte aggregation and activation is probably more complex and could involve several other mediators, such as fibrin degradation products (23), leukotriene $B_4$ (2,24), and platelet activating factor (13, 30). Because of the interrelationship between the coagulation, fibrinolytic, and complement systems, there is every reason to believe that comple-

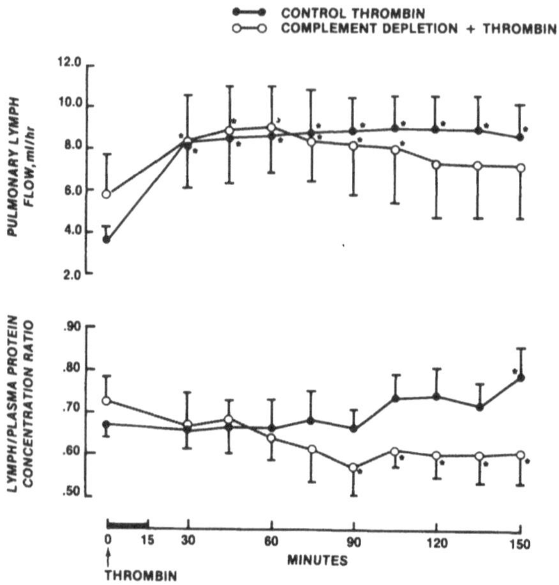


Figure 15

Alterations in pulmonary lymph flow and lymph/ plasma protein concentration ratio after α-thrombin in the control and decomplemented groups.

ment activation after intravascular coagulation is not the only contributing factor to the pulmonary leukostasis and subsequent pulmonary microvascular injury.

Nevertheless, the complement depletion and fibrinolytic inhibition experiments indicate that both fibrinolytic and complement pathways are important in the mediation of lung vascular injury after intravascular coagulation. Both pathways are activated after intravascular coagulation (19, 22, 26), but little is known about the detailed activation processes in intact animals. Activation of the complement pathway releases complement-derived peptides (C3a and C5a) which are hightly chemotactic agents (18, 29), and initiates leukocyte aggregation and activation. The plasminogen system directly activates the complement proteins (22, 26), and this might be the initiating step for complement activation after thrombin.

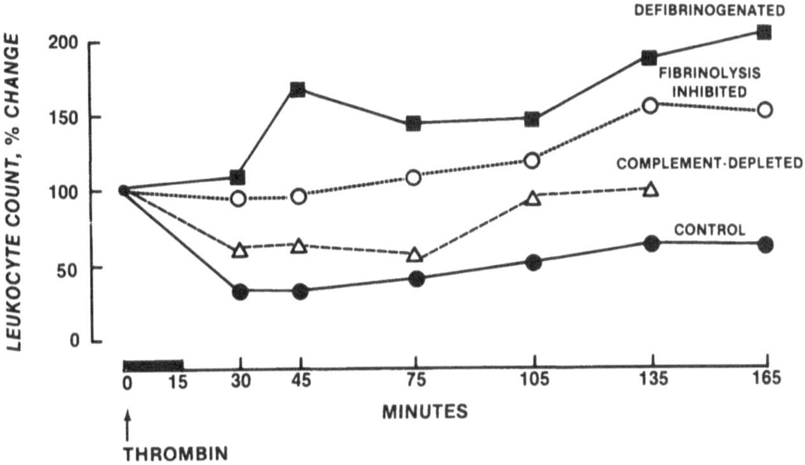


Figure 16.

Changes in leukocyte counts in the control and the various treated groups.

Alternatively, α-thrombin may become actively entrapped in the fibrin clot, where it is retained or degrades into non-clotting thrombin forms. The generation of plasmin readily releases entrapped thrombin forms (8, 31). Both α- and γ-thrombins are known to have potent factor D activity in the alternate complement pathway (5) and could augment complement-dependent processes. In addition various thrombin forms are themselves potent chemotaxins (5).

## 4. Conclusions

Figure 16 summarizes the importance of leukocytes in the mediation of the increased lung vascular permeability after thrombin. The leukocyte counts decreased immediately after infusion of thrombin in control sheep, but the decreases were either transient or non-existent with the interventions that

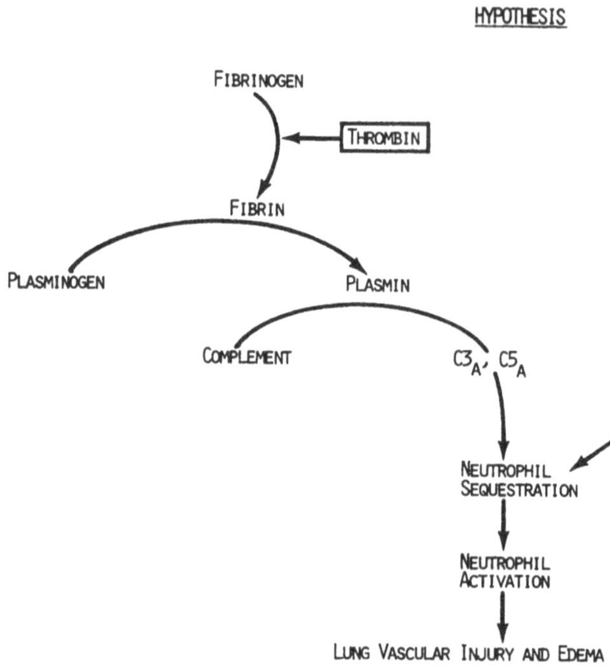


Figure 17

Hypothesis of the mechanism of lung vascular injury following intravascular coagulation with thrombin

prevented the increased permeability. Therefore, the initial decrease in the leukocyte count appears to be a good predictor fo the thrombin-induced lung vascular injury.

In our working hypothesis (Fig. 17), α-thrombin proteolytically converts clottable fibrinogen to fibrin, and the deposition of intravascular fibrin clots entraps α-thrombin. Subsequent activation of plasminogen may directly activate the complement system, resulting in the formation of chemotactic and leukocyte-activating peptides ($C3_a$ and $C5_a$), which induce neutrophil sequestration and activation in pulmonary vessels and subsequent vascular injury. Fibrinolysis also release clot entrapped thrombin forms, which may augment complement activation and may also act as chemotaxins. Other factors generated by fibrinolytic activation (e.g., fibrin degradation products, leukotriene B4, thromboxane A2, platelet activating factor) may directly increase lung vascular permeability or induce further leukocyte aggregation and activation, and thus also contribute to thrombin-induced pulmonary microvascular injury.

ACKNOWLEDGEMENTS

Supported, in part, by NIH HL-17355 and HL-26551. A. Johnson, Ph. D. and J. Cooper, M.D. are postdoctoral fellows (HL-07529). F.L. Minnear, Ph. D., is recipient of a New Investigator Research Award (HL-29273). We would like to acknowledge the technical assistance of Nancy Gertzberg, Charles Kivlen, Linda Lai, Julia Chen, and Lori Hill, and the secretarial assistance of Kathleen Roche. We also appreciate the use of Dr. Kevin Barron's Electron Microscopy Facilities at the Albany Veteran's Administration Hospital.

REFERENCES

1. Bell WR, Shapiro SS, Martinez J, Nossel HJ. The effects of Ancrod, the coagulating enzyme from the venom of the Malayan Pit Viper (A. rhodostoma) on prothrombin and fibrinogen metabolism and fibirn peptide A release in man. J Lab Clin Med 1978; 91:592-604.
2. Bizios R, Minnear FL, van der Zee H, Malik AB. Effect of cyclooxygenase and lipoxygenase inhibition on lung fluid balance after thrombin. J Appl Physiol 1982; 55:462-471.
3. Brigham KL, Woolverton WC, Blake JH, Staub NC. Increased sheep lung vascular permeability caused by Pseudomonas bacteremia. J Clin Invest 1974; 54: 792-804.
4. Del Maestro RF, Thaw HH, Bjork J, Planker M, Arfors KE. Free radicals as mediators of tissue injury. Acta Physiol. Scand 1980; 492:43-57.
5. Fenton JW. Thrombin specificity. New York Acad Sci 1981; 370:468-495.
6. Flick MR, Hoeffel JM, Staub NC. Superoxide dismutase combined with heparin prevents increased lung vascular permeability during lung vascular permeability during air microembolization in sheep. J Appl Physiol 1983. In press.
7. Flick MR, Perel A, Staub NC. Leukocytes are required for increased lung vascular permeability after microembolization in sheep. Circ Res 1981; 48:344-351.
8. Frances CW, Markham RE Jr, Barlow GH, Florack TM, Dobrzynski DM, Marder VJ. Thrombin activity of fibrin thrombi and soluble plasmic derivatives. J Lab Clin Med 1983; 102:220-230.

9. Johnson A, Blumenstock FA, Malik AB. Effect of complement depletion

10. Johnson A, Malik AB. Effect of defibrinogenation on lung fluid and protein exchange after glass bead embolization. J Appl Physiol 1982; 53:895-900.

11. Johnson A, Tahamont MV, Malik AB. Thrombin induced lung vascular injury; Role of fibrinogen and fibrinolysis. Am Rev Resp Dis 1983; 128:38-44.

12. Johnson A, Tahamont MV, Kaplan JE, Malik AB. Effects of pulmonary embolization induced by thrombin and fibrin microaggregates on lung fluid balance. J Appl Physiol 1982; 52:1565-1570.

13. Jin AH, Merton DR, Gorman RR. Acetyl glyceryl ether phosphorylcholine stimulates leukotriene $B_4$ synthesis in human polymorphonuclear leukocytes. J Clin Invest 1982; 70:1058-1065.

14. Malik AB, van der Zee H. Lung vascular permeability following progressive embolization. J Appl Physiol 1978; 45:590-597.

15. Malik AB, Pulmonary microembolism. Physiological Reviews 1983; 63:1114-1207.

16. Minnear FL, Martin D, Taylor AE, Malik AB. Large increase in pulmonary lymph flow after thrombin-induced intravascular coagulation. Fed Proc 1983; 42:1274.

17. MoCostabella PM, Lundquist O, Kapanci Y, Saldeen T. Increased vascular permeability in the delayed microembolism syndrome. Microvasc Res 1978; 15:275-286.

18. Mueller-Eberhard HI, Schreber RD. Molecular biology and chemistry of the alternate pathway of complement. Adv in Immunol 1980; 129:1-53.

19. Mulleretz J. The fibrinolytic system. Scand J Haemt 1979; 34:15-34.

20. O'Brodovitch H, Andrews M, Coates G. Assessment of the coagulation cascade during air microembolization of the sheep and dog lung. Am Rev Resp Dis 1983; 127:(Abst):309.

21. Petrone WF, English DK, Wong K, Malone JM. Free radicals and inflammation: Superoxide dependent activation of a neutrophil chemotactic factor in plasma. Proc Nat'l Acad Sci 1980; 77:1159-1163.

22. Ryan GB. Inflammation and localization of infection. Surg Clin N.A. 1976; 56:831-846.

23. Saldeen T. The microembolism syndrome. In: Microembolism Syndrome, edited by T Saldeen. Stockholm: Almqvist and Wiksell International 1979; pp. 7-44.

24. Samuelsson B. Leukotrienes: Mediators of immediate hypersensitivity reactions and inflammation. Science 1983; 220:568-575.

25. Staub NC. Pulmonary edema. Physiol Rev 1974; 54:678-811.

26. Stormorhen H. Interrelations between the coagulation, fibrinolytic and the kallikrein-kinin system. Scnad J Haem (Suppl.) 1979; 34:24-27.

27. Tahamont MV, Malik AB. Granulocytes mediate the increase in pulmonary vascular permeability after thrombin embolism J Appl Physiol 1983; 54:1489-1495.

28. Taylor AE, Parker JC, Granger DM, Mortillaro NA. Assessment of capillary permeability using lymphatic protein flux; Estimation of the osmotic reflection coefficient. In: The Microcirculation, edited by AE Taylor. New Yrok Academic Press 1981; pp. 19-32.

29. Weissman G, Smolen JE, Korclak HM. Release of inflammatory mediators from stimulated neutrophils. New Eng J Med 1980; 303:27-34.

30. Vaage J. Intravascular platelet aggregation and pulmonary injury. Ann N Y Acad Sci 1982; 384:301-318.

31. Wilner GD, Danitz MP, Mudd MS, Hsieh, K-h, Fenton JW. II. Selective immobilization of α-thrombin by surface-bound fibrin. J Lab Clin Med 1981; 97:403-411.

# THROMBOXANE $A_2$ AS A MECHANISM OF NEUTROPHIL AND LEUKOTRIENE INDUCED LUNG PERMEABILITY

WILLIAM V. HUVAL, M.D., SAMUEL J. DURHAM, SHLOMO LELCUK, M.D., AND HERBERT B. HECHTMAN, M.D.

Department of Surgery
Brigham and Women's Hospital
and
Harvard Medical School;
Boston, MA, USA

## INTRODUCTION

Studies of experimental acid aspiration in dogs have demonstrated that one to two hours after the introduction of acid, white blood cells are sequestered in the lungs. At this same time edema fluid begins to issue from the endotracheal tube (5). An infusion of the cyclo-oxygenase inhibitor, ibuprofen, or the thromboxane (Tx) synthetase inhibitor, ketoconazole, will prevent leukocyte entrapment as well as significantly reduce the volume of edema fluid (1,4). In another experimental setting where complement is activated, $TxA_2$ has been shown to be related to increased capillary permeability in the lungs. Thus, following an infusion of zymosan activated plasma in sheep, leukocyte entrapment in the lungs was associated with an increase in lymph flow and lymph albumin clearance. These changes in the flow and composition of lymph were prevented by infusing the Tx synthetase inhibitor, imidazole (2). We postulate that $TxA_2$ is central in the mechanism of these permeability changes.

Experiments were designed to test whether edema fluid following acid aspiration could induce microvascular permeability when injected into a guinea pig skin bioassay system, and whether this permeability could be altered by inhibition of leukotrienes (LT) or $TxA_2$. We postulate that LT are important intermediaries in the induction of edema, ant that they express their permeability via $TxA_2$ formation. Therefore, a complementary study was done to test the vasotoxicity of pure $LTC_4$ and $LTD_4$ in the bioassay system, and the ability of $TxA_2$ inhibition to modify this LT induced permeability.

## METHODS

Anesthetized, intubated dogs (n=3), on a volume cycled ventilator were aspirated with 0.1 N HCl, 3 ml/kg. The lungs were hyperventilated just after the acid was introduced via a small catheter located just above the carina. Edema fluid was noted after 2 h. It was collected using a trap bottle connected via a "T" piece to the endotracheal tube. The fluid was held for 1h before freezing at -20° C. It was then stored for one to two months until the permeability bioassay was performed.

Permeability assays were performed using male Hartley strain guinea pigs (Elms Hill Farms, Chelmsford, MA) weighing between 35-450 grams. The animals were anesthetized with sodium pentobarbital (50 mg/kg) and the left jugular vein was exposed through a cut-down and cannulated. The back was shaved to allow visualization of the injection sites. Animals selected at random were treated with either the Tx synthetase inhibitor, imidazole (25 mg/kg IV bolus), or the $LTC_4$ and $LTD_4$ receptor antagonist FPL 55712 (Fissons Lab, Leicesteshire, England) administered as a 1 mg/kg IV bolus, followed by an intravenous infusion of 10 μg/kg•min. A total volume of. 0.5 ml saline was used to administer each agent. In untreated control guinea pigs 0.3 ml of normal saline was used to flush the jugular cannulae following insertion.

Twenty minutes after infusion of the antagonists, test substances were injected intradermally with a 27 gauge needle such that a wheal was raised at each site. All injections contained a volume of 0.1 ml and eight sites were used in each guinea pig. The following substances were injected: normal saline, histamine phosphate (1.0 μg/ml), pulmonary edema fluid collected from aspirated dogs (diluted 1:10 with normal saline) and $LTC_4$ and $LTD_4$ (Merck Frosst Canada, Inc.) (50 ng/ml). Ten minutes after the intradermal injections, 10 mg/kg Evan's blue dye contained in 0.1 ml was administered intravenously. The dye was allowed to equilibrate for 15 min. The animals were then killed with a lethal dose of potassium chloride. The dorsal skin containing the injection sites was dissected free. The degree of bluing present on the undersurface of the injection site was then determined in a blinded fashion by three observers using a scale of zero (0) to four (4). A score of zero indicated the absence of bluing, while a score of four was equal to intensity of bluing noted with the injection of 1.0 μg/ml of histamine. Results are reported as the mean and standard error. Groups were compared using a non-paired Student's t-test. Significance was accepted if $p < 0.05$.

## RESULTS

The bioassay sites were calibrated by noting the minimal, zero score of bluing after an injection of saline, and the extreme of 4.0 coloration after histamine injection. Edema fluid diluted 10:1 led to a bluing score of $2.1 \pm 0.2$ units, which was reduced if the LT receptor antagonist FPL 55712 or the Tx synthetase inhibitor was given to the guinea pig ($p < 0.05$, Table 1). The fact that $LTC_4$ and $LTD_4$ led to enhanced microvascular permeability via $TxA_2$ synthesis was seen by the ability of imidazole to reduce the amount of bluing ($p < 0.05$). The ability of FPL 55712 to block $LTC_4$/$LTD_4$ induced permeability is also demonstrated ($p < 0.05$) (Table I).

## DISCUSSION

These results show that the edema which forms after acid aspiration contains a LT which can indirectly provoke microvascular permeability via $TxA_2$ synthesis. The fact that the edema fluid was held for at least 1 h before freezing, and an additional 30 min before bioassay, indicates that neither unstable oxygen-free radicals nor the short lived $TxA_2$, both possibly formed in the aspirated dog, were responsible for the increased permeability in the guinea pigs. The thesis that LT were active intermediaries carried in the edema fluid is supproted by the ability of the LT receptor antagonist FPL 55712 to decrease permeability. Of most interest is the ability to reduce the permeability potential of both edema fluid as well as $LTC_4$ and $LTD_4$ by blocking $TxA_2$ synthesis.

Other reports have shown that LT express their vasospasitity via $TxA_2$ synthesis (3). It now appears that LT vasotoxicity is mediated, at least in part, by LT induced $TxA_2$ synthesis. The fact that inhibition of Tx in the intact aspirated animal also prevents leukosequestration in the lungs implies that this prostanoid may also mediate chemotaxis (1).

TABLE I

| TEST AGENT | NO. ANIMALS | GUINEA PIG TREATMENT | BLUING |
|---|---|---|---|
| Saline | 8 | None | 0 |
| Histamine | 5 | None | $4.0 \pm 0.1$ |
| Edema Fluid | 9 | None | $2.1 \pm 0.2$ |
| | 6 | FPL 55712 | $1.4 \pm 0.2^*$ |
| | 5 | Imidazole | $0.8 \pm 0.2^*$ |
| $LTC_4/LTD_4$ | 14 | None | $2.0 \pm 0.1$ |
| | 6 | FPL 55712 | $0.4 \pm 0.1^\dagger$ |
| | 11 | Imidazole | $1.0 \pm 0.1^\dagger$ |

* $p < 0.05$ with respect to edema fluid injection sites of non-treated group

† $p < 0.05$ with respect to $LTC_4/LTD_4$ injection sites of non-treated group

SUMMARY

Experimental acid aspiration leads to leukosequestration in the lungs and permeability edema which can be attenuated by inhibiting thromboxane (Tx) $A_2$. The intermediate involvement of leukotriene (LT) $C_4$ and $D_4$ was tested using a guinea pig skin bioassay of permeability. Edema fluid from acid aspirated dogs led to marked skin permeability in the guinea pig which could be significantly reduced by inhibiting guinea pig LT receptors with FPL 55712 or $TxA_2$ synthetase with imidazole. Further, the permeability induced by pure $LTC_4$ and $LTD_4$ injected into guinea pig skin could be modified with imidazole ($p < 0.05$). These data indicate that inflammatory reactions in the lungs can provoke the release of LT and that these agents can act by stimulating $TxA_2$ synthesis, which in turn leads to microvascular permeability.

## REFERENCES

1. Huval WV, Dunham BM, Lelcuk S, Valeri CR, Shepro D, Hechtman HB. Thromboxane mediation of cardiovascular dysfunction following aspiration. Surgery (In press).

2. Krausz MM, Utsunomiya T, Dunham B, Valeri CR, Shepro D, Hechtman HB. Inhibition of permeability edema with imidazole. Surgery 1982; 92:299-308.

3. Piper PJ, Samhoun MN. Stimulation of arachidonic acid metabolites and generation of thromboxane $A_2$ by leukotrienes $B_4$, $C_4$ and $D_4$ in guinea-pig lung in-vitro. Br J Pharm. 1982; 77:267-275.

4. Utsunomiya T, Krausz MM, Shepro D, Hechtman HB. Treatment of aspiration pneumonia with ibuprofen and prostacyclin ($PGI_2$). Surgery 1981; 90:170-176.

5. Utsunomiya T, Krausz MM, Dunham B, Valeri CR, Levine L, Shepro D, Hechtman HB. Modification of the inflammatory response to aspiration with ibuprofen. Am J Physiol. 1982; 243:H903-H910.

## ACKNOWLEDGEMENTS

Supported in part by The National Institute of Health, Grants No. GM24891-05, The U.S. Army Medical Research and Development Command, Contract No. DAMD17-78-C-8026; The Brigham Surgical Group, Inc. and The Trauma Research Foundation. Address all Correspondence to: Herbert B. Hechtman, M.D. Brigham and Women's Hospital, 75 Frances Street, Boston, MA 02115, USA.

# PATHOPHYSIOLOGY AND TREATMENT OF PULMONARY AIR EMBOLISM IN SHEEP

NORMAN V. STAUB, KURT H. ALBERTINE AND
PEGGY CULVER

Cardiovascular Research Institute and
Departments of Physiology and Anatomy
University of California, San Francisco,
San Francisco, CA 94143, USA

In many kinds of acute lung injury, there is an increase in the pulmonary vascular resistance and pathologic evidence of multiple pulmonary emboli. Some workers feel that the microemboli are an important, if not the principal, cause of the lung injury which may progress to Adult Respiratory Distress Syndrome (ARDS) (19,23).

In the last several years, my associates and I have found that several kinds of foreign material will produce acute microembolism lung injury in sheep. We and others have used mineral oil, glass microspheres and thrombin infusions to produce the embolization (12, 14).

We are now using air microemboli exclusively. Air emboli are a clinical problem in diving medicine (5), in neurosurgery (17) and in other clinical conditions (7). For use in unanesthetized sheep, air emboli are nearly ideal because they cause a highly reproducible, completely reversible injury that is confines to the pulmonary microcirculation (15). Thus, air microembolization is our paradigm for the acute microembolization syndrome.

In the awake sheep, which has been suitably instrumented for the measurement of pulmonary hemodynamics and lung lymph dynamics (15, 21), we infuse air emboli, approximately 1 mm diamter, into the right atrium or pulmonary artery at the rate of 2-3 ml/(kg x h) continuously for up to 4h. Figure 1 shows the time course of one experiment to illustrate the major features. Before embolization, the hemodynamic and lymph dynamic variables are stable (first 2h). With the onset of the embolization, of the embolization, of course, pulmonary arterial pressure and calculated pulmonary resistance increased significantly due both to physical obstruction by the emboli and to active vasoconstriction (lung lymph concentration of thromboxane $B_2$ (metabolite of thromboxane $A_2$) increased markedly). Since the air in the bubbles is under pressure in small pulmonary arteries and arterioles, it escapes into the alveolar gas and the bubbles shrink and disappear. That is why continuous a infusion of air is necessary to maintain the obstruction. During embolization,

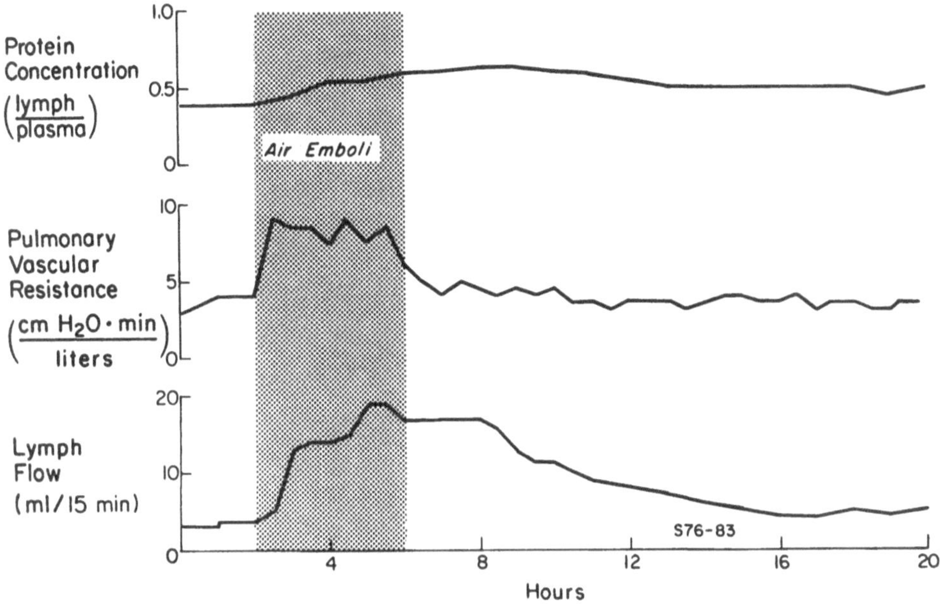


Figure 1

Time course (20h) of lung lymph flow and lymph protein concentration in response to intravenous air embolism in an unanesthetized sheep. Emboli were infused from the second to the sixth hour to increase pulmonary vascular resistance approximately twofold. Lymph flow increased within the first hour, peaking in the fourth hour at about five times baseline flow. The lymph/plasma protein concentration ratio also increased modestly. When the air embolization was stopped, the pulmonary vascular resistance decreased to near baseline level within 2h. Lymph flow remained elevated, however, returning slowly to the baseline level over the next 12h with a half time of 4-1/2h.

lung lymph flow increases to levels 3-5 times the baseline level reaching a quasi-stable condition after about 2-3h. This large increase in lymph flow occurs even though a large fraction of the pulmonary vascular bed is obstructed by emboli, thus decreasing the surface area for liquid exchange. In addition, the lymph to plasma protein concentration ratio (L/P) remains near or at the baseline level.

When the embolization ends, the pulmonary artery pressure

and calculated vascular resistance decreased to normal, usually within 1-2h. But lung lymph flow remained elevated for a prolonged period, slowly returning to normal over 24h.

As Ohkuda and associates showed (15) the injury caused by the air emboli increases both lung microvascular filtration rate and the rate of protein leakage. This is most conveniently expressed as the lymph protein clearance (lymph flow x L/P), which I will use in this chapter as our index of microvascular permeability change. This is an important point because lymph flow and protein leakage are also affected by microvascular hydrostatic pressure, which is clearly elevated during the microembolism experiments. Therefore, the lymph protein clearance has to be related to some controlled variable. We have chosen to relate the lymph protein clearance to the calculated pulmonary vascular resistance. This allows us to correct for changes in lung hemodynamics, which can sometimes complicate the interpretation of lung lymph data.

## PATHOGENESIS

Since we have published all of our depletion studies (1,2,6) I will only summarize them. We found that depletion of circulating fibrinogen (using pit viper venom) or platelets (using specific anti-serum) had no detectable effect on the time course or severity of the lung injury caused by microemboli, as judged by lymph protein clearance.

Recently, O'Brodovich and his associates (13) studied the coagulation cascade during air microembolization in unanesthetized sheep. Although they limited the duration of air embolization to 30 min, the expected elevation in pulmonary artery pressure and the marked decrease in systemic arterial oxygen tension occurred. But they did not detect any decrease in radioactively-labeled plasma fibrinogen levels. When they infused thrombin intravenously, however, plasma fibrinogen levels fell promptly. Thus, fibrin deposition may be central to microemboli due to intravascular clotting but it is not necessarily involved in acute microembolism lung injury, in general.

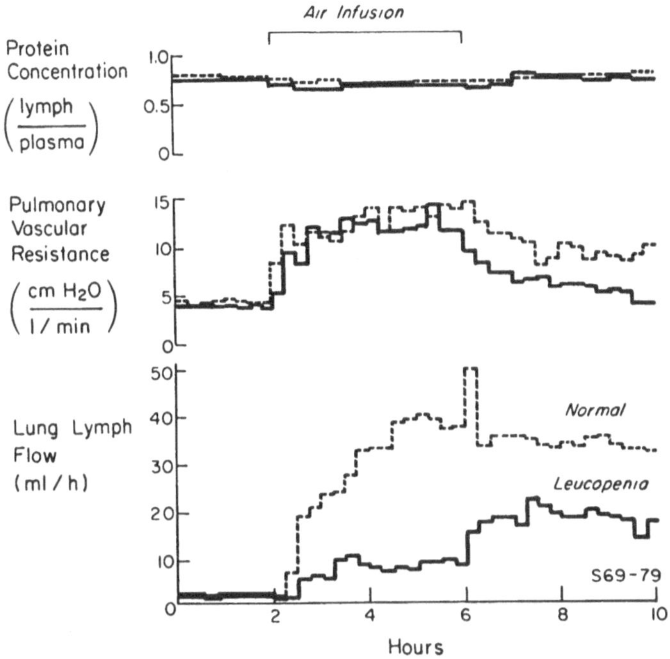


Figure 2

Two experiments in an unanesthetized sheep to show the marked attenuating effect of leucopenia on the air embolism lung injury (From reference 6 by permission).

When we made sheep leucopenic, using nitrogen mustard, the air embolism response was attenuated. An example is shown in Figure 2. These results indicated that some function of leucocytes (most likely the polymorphonuclear leucocytes) was involved in the pathogenesis of the endothelial injury.

We have quantified the effects of air emboli within the pulmonary microcirculation (22). The air bubbles embolize small pulmonary arteries, then move into arterioles as pulmonary arterial pressure increases and as the air within the bubbles escapes. The most striking feature is the accumulation of leucocytes at the embolus-blood interface, as shown in Figure 3.

When the air emboli are completely reabsorbed (none pass through the pulmonary capillaries), residual leucocyte emboli can be found lodged in terminal arterioles. On close inspection, the cells at the air-blood interface are predominantly polymorphonuclear leucocytes, although a few lymphocytes and platelets are also found there (22).

In the last two years, we have examined the ultrastructural basis for the microvascular injury. The injury consists of intercellular gap formation or necrosis of portions of endothelial cells and disruption of their basal laminae in the small pulmonary arteries, as shown in Figure 4. Neutrophils

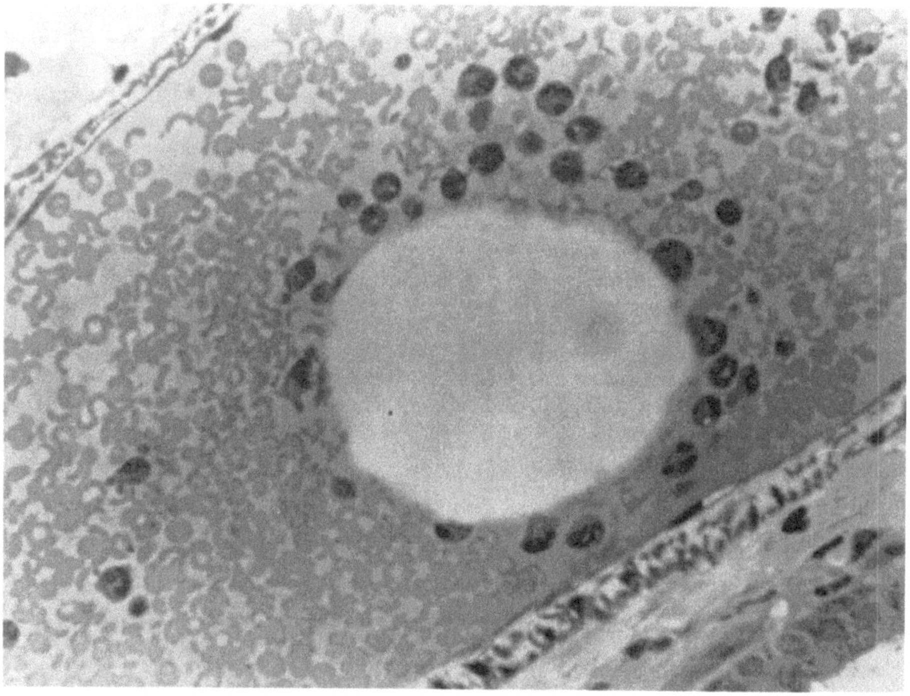

Figure 3

Histologic section showing an air bubble wedged in a small pulmonary artery (note smooth muscle in vessel wall). Numerous leucocytes surround the embolus-blood interface (mostly polymorphonuclear leucocytes.

are frequently associated with the lesions. There was no evidence of any deposition of fibrin.

Quantitatively, all of the ultrastructurally-detectable injury was confined to the small pulmonary arteries and

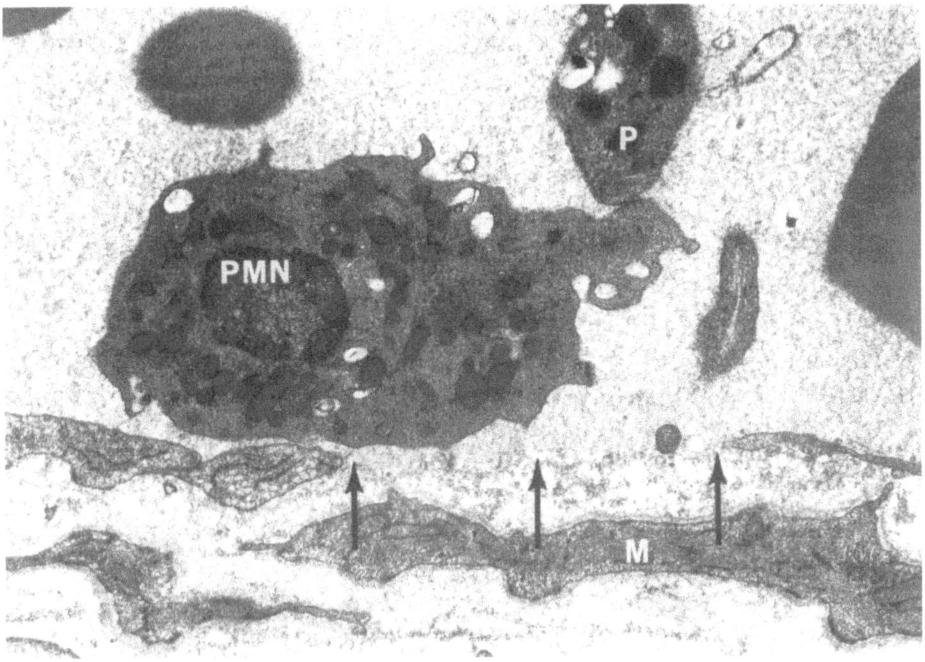


Figure 4

Electron microscopic picture of the wall of a small pulmonary arteriole (smooth muscle cell, M). The endothelium is disrupted over a distance of approximately 3 um (arrows). Adjacent to the injury is a polymorphonuclear leucocyte (PMN) and a platelet (P). 17,000X.

arterioles, as summarized in Table I. This suggests that the rate of liquid and protein leakage will be sensitive to pulmonary arterial pressure.

## TREATMENT

In the empirical treatment of acute lung injury, high dose corticosteroids (30 mg/kg) have been shown to have a protective effect against microembolic and septic lung injury (3, 16, 20, 23). But there is no consensus about whether corticosteroids are useful in their treatment (that is, after the injury has occurred). We have studied the effects of corticosteroids as a prevention and as an early treatment of air embolism lung injury in six sheep.

Figure 5 shows the time course of lung lymph dynamics and pulmonary vascular resistance in one sheep on two occasions;

TABLE I

SITES OF ENDOTHELIAL INJURY IN LUNG
FOLLOWING INTRAVENOUS AIR EMBOLI IN SHEEP

| Condition | No. | Arterioles* | Capillaries | Venules |
|---|---|---|---|---|
| Control | 2 | 0/28+ | 0/200 | 0/15 |
| Air Emboli | 4 | 52/52 | 0/400 | 2/46 |

* Arterioles and venules include vessels between 30-50 um diameters. Capillaries are 8-10 um diameter alveolar wall vessels.

\+ Number of vessels with lesions/total vessels examined.

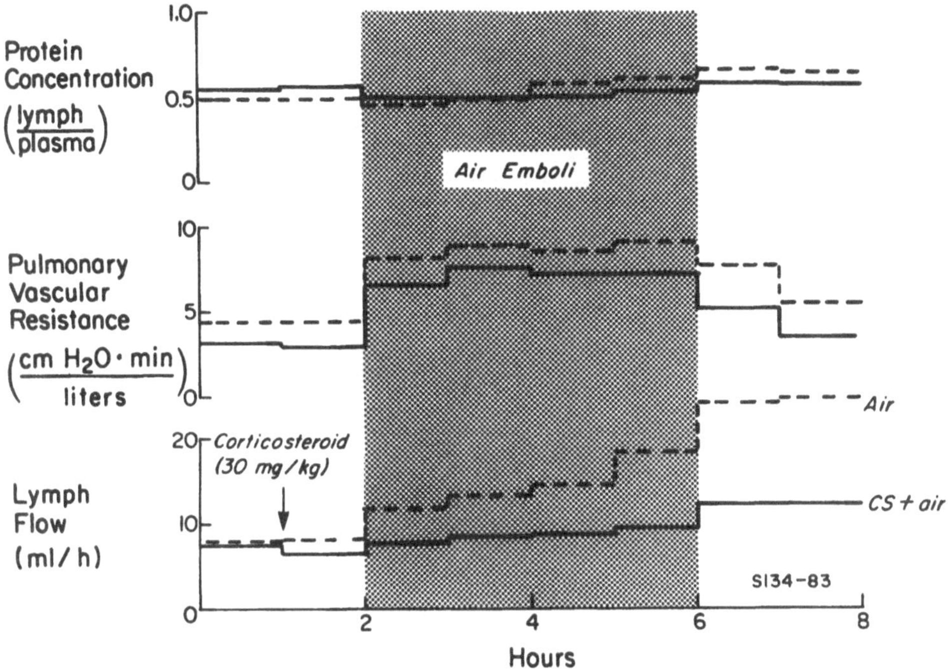


Figure 5

Two experiments in an unanesthetized sheep showing the effect of high dose corticosteroids in preventing lung injury during microembolization. The lymph flow response to embolization is markedly attenuated.

when air was infused alone and when methylprednisolone (30 mg/kg) was given intravenously one hour before the onset of air embolization. The major effect is on the lung lymph flow which is only slightly increased above the baseline level.

Figure 6 shows the time course of two experiments in the same sheep as in Figure 5. In this instance, however, the corticosteroid was injected after one hour of air embolization. Following the corticosteroid treatment, lymph flow is significantly less than with the air emboli alone, although not so low as when the corticosteroid was given as a prevention.

Figure 7 summarizes the lymph protein clearance as a function of the pulmonary vascular resistance, which corrects for the slight vasodilation caused by the corticosteroid. Corticosteroid prevention eliminated nearly all of the increase in pro-

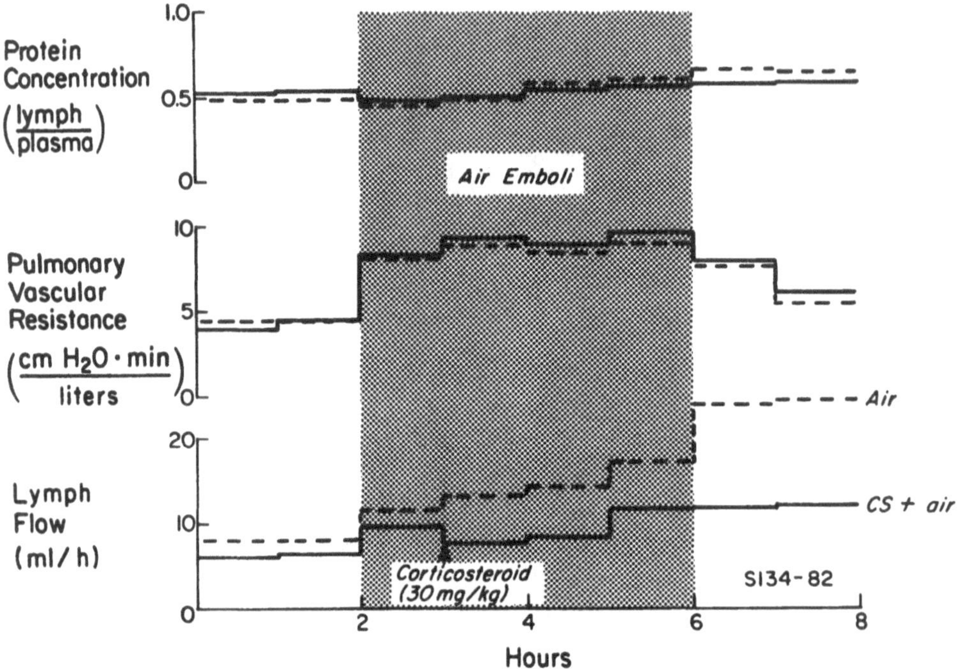


Figure 6

Two experiments in an unanesthetized sheep showing the effect of high dose corticosteroids as an early treatment (1h after the onset of air embolization). The lymph flow response is reduced, although not as markedly with corticosteroid prevention. Data from the same animal was used for Figures 5 and 6.

tein clearance, and early treatment also attenuated the increase in protein clearance.

We are continuing these investigations along two lines. We are quantifying the ultrastructural effects of air emboli when corticosteroids are given. In two studies completed using corticosteroid prevention, we have found that methylprednisolone prevents the attachment of neutrophils to the air emboli as well as markedly decreases the number of endothelial lesions in the small pulmonary arteries and arterioles. Secondly, we have begun to study the effect of late treatment with corticosteroid. In one completed experiment, we gave steroids every 6h for 24h beginning at the fourth hour of air embolization. Although there was no immediate effect, there was a faster recovery time course following cessation of air embolization.

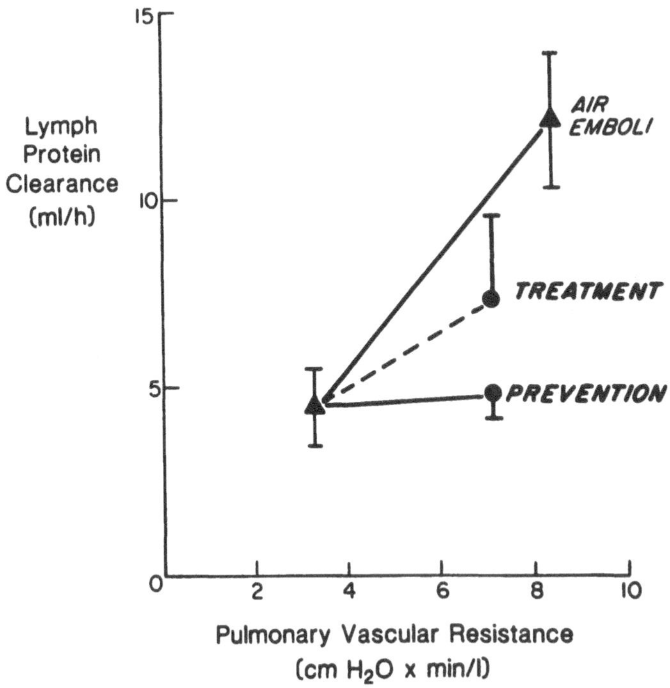


Figure 7

Summary of all experiments in six sheep comparing high dose corticosteroid prevention and treatment of air embolization lung injury. The lymph protein clearance is plotted as a function of calculated pulmonary vascular resistance. This corrects for hemodynamic changes which may occur during treatment. Corticosteroid prevention eliminated the increase in lymph protein clearance. As an early treatment, the high dose corticosteroid was partially effective. Data are shown as mean $\pm$ one standard deviation.

We conclude that, although corticosteroids are not able to reverse injury that has already occurred, they are able to prevent extension of injury. For those comtemplating the use of corticosteroids in patients with acute lung injury, our data indicate that <u>early use will be more beneficial.</u> Any delay in the decision to treat using corticosteroids will reduce their effectiveness. Even though we have completed only one experiment, the corticosteroids appear to have a beneficial effect in speeding recovery from embolic injury. This confirms the report of Cheney and associates (1979) who found corticosteroids to be beneficial in the recovery of goats from oleic acid lung injury.

Another aspect of acute lung injury is the possible role of adrenergic receptors in the regulation of lung liquid balance. Foy and associates (8) showed that isoproterenol (a beta-1 agonist) ameliorated the liquid and protein leakage during pseudomonas bacteremia in awake sheep. They attributed the benefit to a decrease in pulmonary microvascular pressure following vasodilation. On the other hand, Hakim and coworkers (10), reported that beta-receptor blockade by propranolol increased lung lymph and protein flow in anesthetized sheep. They suggested that beta-receptors may control microvascular permeability.

A number of pharmacologists, including Green (9) and Joyner and associates (11) found that beta-agonists will block the permeability-increasing effect of histamine in systemic vascular beds. In the guinea pig, a beta-2 agonist, terbutaline, prevented histamine-induced pulmonary edema (18).

We have examined the effects of continuous infusion of the beta agonist, terbutaline, on the air microembolism lung injury in seven awake sheep. The infusions were made at the rate of.6 ug/(kg x min) beginning 1h before the onset of air embolization. This dose of the beta agonist is sufficient to increase heart rate (beta-1 effect) by 30-50 beats/min.

Figure 8 shows the time course of air embolization in a sheep on two occasions; air emboli alone and during a continuous infusion of the beta-2 agonist terbutaline. The increase in lung lymph flow is significantly attenuated by the beta agonist. In parallel to that, however, is a large decrease in pulmonary vascular resistance.

Figure 9 summarizes the lymph protein clearance data for all of these experiments. The lymph protein clearance was reduced during the beta agonist infusion, but only to the extent that

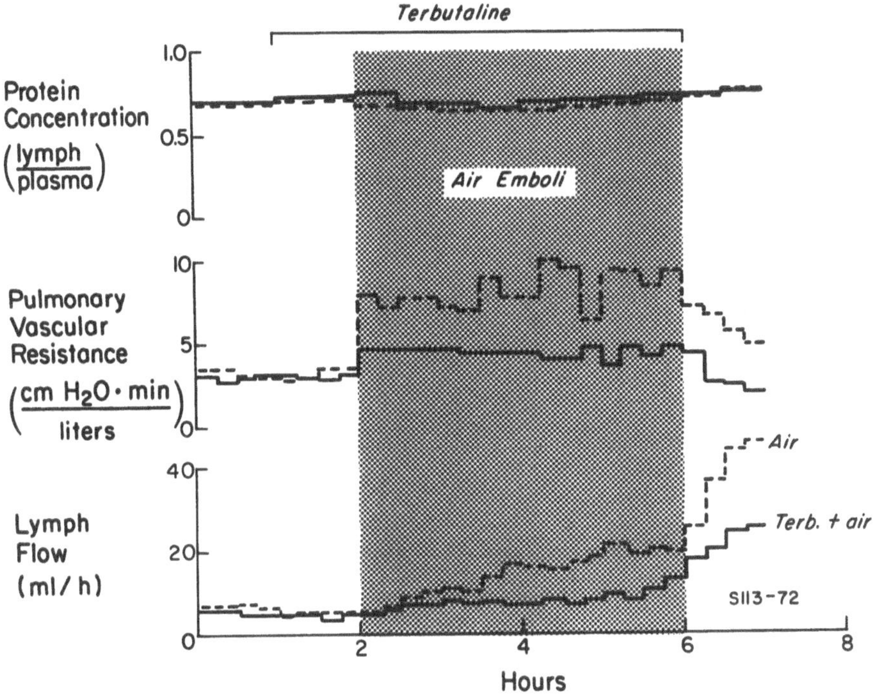


Figure 8

Two experiments in an awake sheep to show the effect of the beta-2 agonist terbutaline on the lung lymph flow and hemodynamic response to air embolization. The beta agonist prevented about half of the rise in pulmonary vascular resistance, indicating that a substantial portion of the increased resistance is due to vasoconstriction rather than obstruction by the air bubbles. Terbutaline also significantly reduced the increase in lung lymph flow.

the pulmonary vascular resistance was decreased.

In three sheep, we gave additional amount of air to increase pulmonary vascular resistance to the same level as with the air emboli alone. When this occurred, the lymph protein clearance increased to the same level as with air emboli alone.

We conclude that any beneficial action of beta receptor stimulation in air embolism lung injury is due to its hemodynamic (vasodilator) effect. Beta receptors have no effect on the microvascular injury.

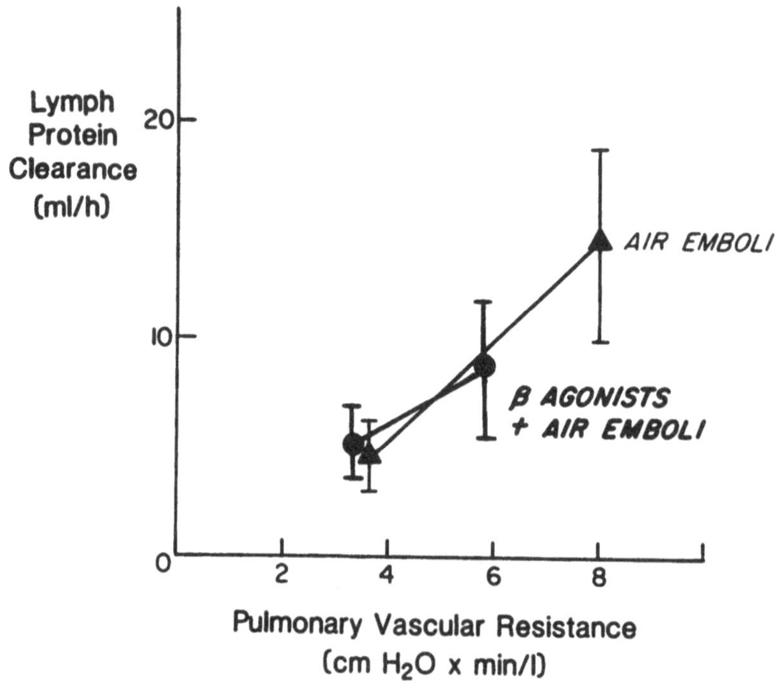


Figure 9

Summary of all experiments in seven sheep using the beta receptor agonist. Although the lymph protein clearance is reduced, it appears to be entirely due to the decrease of pulmonary vascular resistance because the solid circle lies on the line connecting the baseline and air emboli alone points. Data are shown as mean $\pm$ one standard deviation.

## CONCLUSION

We have reviewed the pathophysiology of air microembolism lung injury in unanesthetized sheep. The injury is independent of the clotting cascade and of platelets but is directly dependent on the presence of circulating leucocytes. Pathologically, the injury appears to be mediated by neutrophils, which have become attached (and presumably activated) at the embolus-blood interface. The localization of the injury to the pulmonary arteriolar endothelium is as expected, since that is where the microemboli and neutrophils lodge.

The injury can be largely prevented or attenuated by the use of high dose corticosteroids, among whose functions is that of inhibiting neutrophil aggregation and activation.

Beta adrenergic receptor stimulation has no effect on the time course of lung injury following microembolization, although it attenuates the lymph and protein flow response in parallel to its effects on pulmonary vascular resistance and pulmonary arterial pressure. This type of injury (which is largely an arterial injury) pulmonary vasodilation, with lowering of pulmonary arterial pressure will be beneficial.

## REFERENCES

1. Binder AS, Nakahara K, Ohkuda K, Kageler W, Staub NC. Effect of heparin or fibrinogen depletion on lung fluid balance in sheep after emboli. J Appl Physiol. 1979; 47: 213-219.
2. Binder AS, Kageler W, Perel A, Flick MR, Staub NC. Effect of platelet depletion on lung vascular permeability after microemboli in sheep. J Appl Physiol. 1980; 48:414-420.
3. Cheney FW, Huang TH, Gronka R.. Effects of methylprednisolone on experimental pulmonary injury. Ann Surg. 1979; 190:236-242.
4. Elliot DH, Hallenbeck JM. The pathophysiology decompression sickness. In: The Physiology and Medicine of Diving. (PB Bennett and DH Elliott, eds). Bailliere Tindall, London. 1975; pp 435-455.
5. Flick FR, Perel A, Staub NC. Leucocytes are required for increased lung microvascular permeability after microembolization in sheep. Circ Res. 1981; 48:344-351.
6. Brigham KL, Bowers RE, McKeen CR. Methylprednisolone prevention of increased lung vascular permeability following endotoxemia in sheep. J Clin Invest. 1981; 67: 1103-1110.
7. Clark MC, Flick MR. Permeability pulmonary edema caused by venous air embolism. Am Rev Resp Dis. 1984. In press.
8. Foy T, Marion J, Brigham KL, Harris TR. Isoproterenol and aminophylline reduce lung capillary filtration during high permeability. J Appl Physiol. 1979; 46:146-151.
9. Green KL. The anti-inflammatory effect of catecholamines in the peritoneal cavity and kind paw of the mouse. Brit J Pharmacol. 1972; 45:322-332.
10. Hakim TS, Minnear FL, van der Zee H, Barie PS, Malik AB. Adrenoceptor control of lung fluid and protein exchange. J Appl Physiol. 1981; 51:68-72.
11. Joyner WL, Svensjö E, Arfors KE. Simultaneous measurements

of macromolecular leakage and arteriolar blood flow as altered by PGE1 and beta-2-receptor stimulant in the hamster cheek pouch. Microvasc. 1979; 18:301-310.

12. Malik AB, Johnson A, Tahamont MV. Mechanisms of lung vascular injury after intravascular coagulation. Ann N York Sci. 1982; 384:213-234.

13. O'Brodovich H, Andrew M, Silver R, Coates G. Assessment of the coagulation cascade during air mecroembolism of the lung. J Appl Physiol. 1983. In press.

14. Ohkuda K, Nakahara K, Weidner WJ, Binder A, Staub NC. Lung fluid exchange after uneven pulmonary artery obstruction in sheep. Circulat Res. 1978; 43:152-161.

15. Ohkuda K, Nakahara K, Binder A, Staub NC. Venous air emboli in sheep-reversible increase in lung microvascular permeability. J Appl Physiol. 1981; 51:887-894.

16. Perel M, Flick M, Staub NC. Methylprednisolone partially protects against microemboli induced permeability injury in lungs of awake sheep. Am Rev Resp Dis. 1980; 121:121-442.

17. Perschau RA, Munson ES, Chapin JC. Pulmonary interstitial edema after multiple venous air emboli. Anestheiol. 1976; 45:364-368.

18. Persson CGA, Eyefalt I, Grega GJ, Svensjo E. The role of B-receptor agonists in the inhibition of pulmonary edema. Ann N Y Acad Sci. 1982; 384:544-557.

19. Saldeen T. The microembolism syndrome. Microvasc Res. 1976; 11:227-259.

20. Sibbald WJ, Anderson RR, Reid B, Holliday RL, Driedger AA. Alveolo-capillary permeability in human septic adult respiratory distress syndrome. Effect of high dose corticosteroid therapy. Chest 1981; 79:133-142.

21. Staub NC, Bland RD, Brigham KL, Demling R, Erdmann III AJ, Woolverton WC. Preparation of chronic lung lymph fistulas in sheep. J Surg Res. 1975; 19:315-320.

22. Staub NC, Schultz EL, Albertine KH. Leucocytes and pulmonary microvascular injury. Ann N Y Acad Sci. 1982; 384: 332-342.

23. Wilson JW, Ratcliff NB, Hackel DB. The lung in hemorrhagic shock. Am J Path. 1970; 58:337-352.

# THE PLASMA KALLIKREIN-KININ SYSTEM IN MULTIPLE TRAUMA AND POST-TRAUMATIC SHOCK

ANSGAR O. AASEN, M.D.

Institute for Surgical Research, Rikshospitalet, Oslo 1 and Surgical Department, Ullevaal University Hospital, University of Oslo, Oslo 1, Norway

## INTRODUCTION

In both experimental studies on trauma and severely traumatized patients, activation of the plasma protease systems have been demonstrated. These disturbances of body homeostasis is well known for the coagulation and fibrinolytic system (10,11, 13,24,29,31,36). Furthermore changes in these protease systems have been recognized to be of major pathophysiological significance for development of the microembolism syndrome characterized by acute progressive respiratory distress following trauma (24,29,31,36).

During the last few years activation of the plasma kallikrein-kinin (32,33) and the complement (21) systems have also been reported in this state. The present paper summarizes recent experimental and clinical studies by our group on changes in the plasma kallikrein-kinin system found after trauma.

<u>The plasma kallikrein-kinin system.</u>

In recent years, it has become apparent that the coagulation, fibrinolytic, complement and kallikrein-kinin systems are very closely interrelated (16,30). Furthermore several studies have demonstrated that a common function of these systems is host defence mechanisms against injury.

A key component of these interrelated functions is the Hageman factor (FXII) first described by Ratnoff and Colopy in 1955 (27). Subsequent studies have revealed the importance of this factor for kinin generations (30). A fragment of Hageman factor (FXIIf, fig. 1) is able to convert the proenzyme of the plasma kallikrein-kinin system, prekallikrein, to the active enzyme kallikrein. Upon attacking the substrate high molecular weight kininogen (HMvK) bradykinin is formed. Bradykinin is one of the most potent vasodilating agents hitherto discovered (17), furthermore this substance has strong permeability increasing effects. Besides generating kinins, kallikrein also can induce complement and fibrinolytic activity by activating C1 and plasminogen (30,17).

The activities generated by kallikrein are regulated by natur-

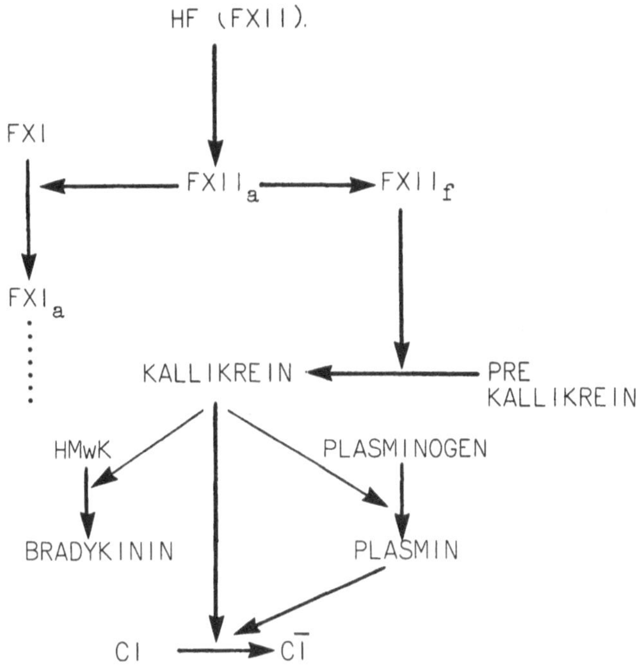


Figure 1

"The plasma kallikrein-kinin system in post-traumatic shock".

The Hageman factor, prekallikrein activation pathways. Abbrievation used, HF, Hageman Factor (FXII), HMwK, high molecular weight Kininogen. C1, the first component of the complement system.

ally occurring protease inhibitors. In human plasma $C^1$-esterase inhibitor and $\alpha_2$-macroglobulin are the most important inhibitors of plasma kallikrein (20,28,34).

Chromogenic peptide substrate assays

Chromogenic peptide substrates (CPS) are small synthetic peptides with the chromophore p-nitroaniline (pNA) coupled to the terminal carboxyl group in an amide linkage (7,8,40,41). These substrates are the basis for a new generation of analyses of serine proteases. The enzymatic cleavage of the peptide-pNA amid linkage in CPS results in release of pNA. This reaction can be monitored at 405 nm in a spectrophotometer, and can easily be automated using equipment found in most clinical chemistry laboratories (2,9).

Assays based on CPS are now developed for determination of active enzyme, proenzyme and functional inhibition of several proteases including components of the plasma kallikrein-kinin system (2).

Two chromogenic peptide substrates are available for determination of components of the plasma kallikrein-kinin system (Table 1).

Experimental post traumatic shock

In a recent study by Saugstad and coworkers (33) lung insufficiency was induced according to the method described by Porcelli et al (26). In this model post traumatic shock is induced by combining hemorrhagic hypotension (50 mm Hg for two hours and clamping of the portal tree for 20 minutes).

In all animals morphological changes in the lung characteristic of post-traumatic lung insufficiency developed (23). Incipient lung changes were recognized as early as 4 hours after initiation of the trauma (23). Perivascular and intraseptal edema, scattered microthrombi and trapping of leucocytes in lung microvessels were the most frequent morphological findings. These changes grew gradually more pronounced towards circulatory collapse. During late stages also interstitial hemorrhages, intraalveolar edema and fibrinoid material were found (23).

| SUBSTRATE | CHEMICAL STRUCTURE | APPLICATIONS |
|---|---|---|
| S-2302[a] | H-D-Pro-Phe-Arg-pNA | Plasma Kallikrein, Prekallikrein, |
| Chromozym-PK[b] | Bz-Pro-Phe-Arg-pNA | Antikallikrein and Kallikrein Activators |

a Made by Kabi Vitrum AB, Stockholm, Sweden.
b Made by Pentapharm AG, Basel, Switzerland.

Table I. Chromogenic peptide substrates available for determination of components of the plasma kallikrein-kinin system

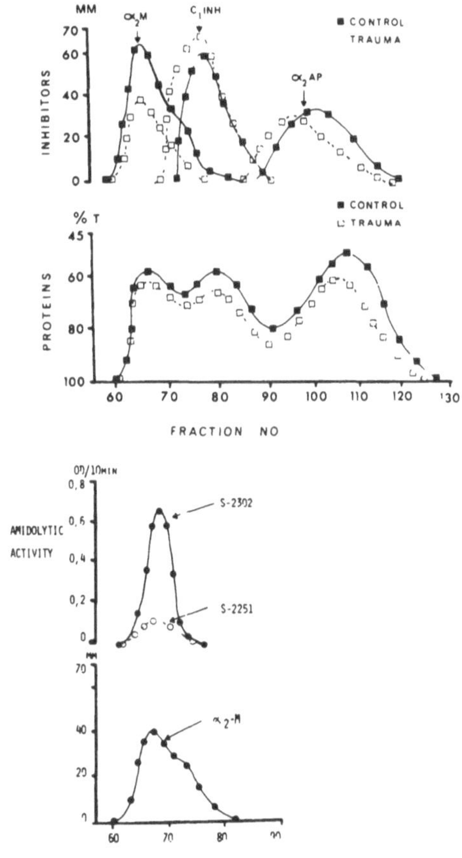


Figure 2

Sephadex G-150 gel filtration of normal plasma and plasma from a patient with multiple trauma. Inhibitor and protein distribution is shown in the upper pannel. In the lower pannel proteolytic activity towards S-2302 (kallikrein) and S-2251 (plasmin) is demonstrated in the $\alpha_2$-macroglobulin containing fractions (From 3 ).

In this model a gradually decrease of plasma prekallikrein developed together with a significant elevation of kallikrein activity (33). These changes were accompanied by a significant reduction of functional kallikrein activity. Also high molecular weight kinogen values gradually decreased reaching 28 % of initial values within 12 hours after the start of the experiments in individual animals (33).

Multiple trauma

In a recent study by our group plasma proteolysis was evaluated in 15 severely injured patients (3). There were 9 survivors and 6 fatal cases. The injuries included multiple fractures and a chest trauma in all cases. Several cases in both groups had flail chest and intraabominal injuries requiring surgical treatment (3).

Immediately after trauma plasma prekallikrein values were significantly reduced both in survivors and fatal cases (3). PKK values, however, were normalized within the first five days after injury in the survivors whereas PKK values were maintained reduced and showed a decreasing pattern in the fatal cases (3). Functional plasma kallikrein inhibition values were found within the normal range during the first week after injury in both groups of patients.

Evidence for kallikrein activation was obtained by gel-filtration of plasma from these patients. As shown in fig. 2, three protein peaks were obtained. In column fractions containing $\alpha_2$ macroglobulin proteolytic activity largely towards S-2302 was found. This demonstrate the formation of $\alpha_2$-macroglobulin kallikrein complexes in the patient. In these traumatized patients also Hageman factor values were significantly reduced when compared with normals in both groups of patients on the first day after injury (3). During the first week after trauma, Hageman factor values were normalized in the survivors whereas this parameter remained reduced in the fatal cases.

These changes of the plasma kallikrein-kinin system is further demonstrated in the following two case reports.

Case report 1

A fifty year old female was admitted to our hospital after a fall into the street from the third floor. She had multiple complicated fractures in both feet and ankles, fractures in both forearms and multiple rib fractures. Shortly after admission her Hb concentrations fell from 11,9 gm/100 ml to 8,5 gm/100 ml. Explorative laparotomy disclosed a large retroperitoneal bleeding. During the first few days in the intensive care unit, the patient developed severe respiratory distress. Her platelets number fell, Normotest® values were prolonged, arterial oxygen tension reduced, and arterial $CO_2$ values raised (fig. 3). The condition was recognized as posttraumatic lung insufficiency. She received Macrodex 70 and steroids i.v. and on the fourth day respirator treatment with positive end-expiratory pressure was started. Subsequently her clinical condition greatly improved, the platelet number was normalized (fig. 3 ), and she was taken off the respirator after nine days.

Reduced prekallikrein values were found immediately after admission (fig. 4). PKK values, however, markedly increased during respirator treatment as her condition improved (fig. 4). Also functional kallikrein inhibition values increased during this initial phase of treatment. During the second week of treatment the patient developed severe infections of the complicated fractures in her feet. She was treated with antibiotics, but finally her left foot had to be amputated. Postoperatively she got pneumonia and died shortly after the operation.

During this period of the treatment the patient revealed a decreasing pattern of PKK values (fig. 4).

Case report 2

A sixty year old female was hospitalized after a traffic accident. Her injuries included brain contusion, three rib fractures with contution of the lung, a fracture of the right leg, multiple fractures in the pelvis and rupture of the urinary bladder. Immediately after admittance the bladder-

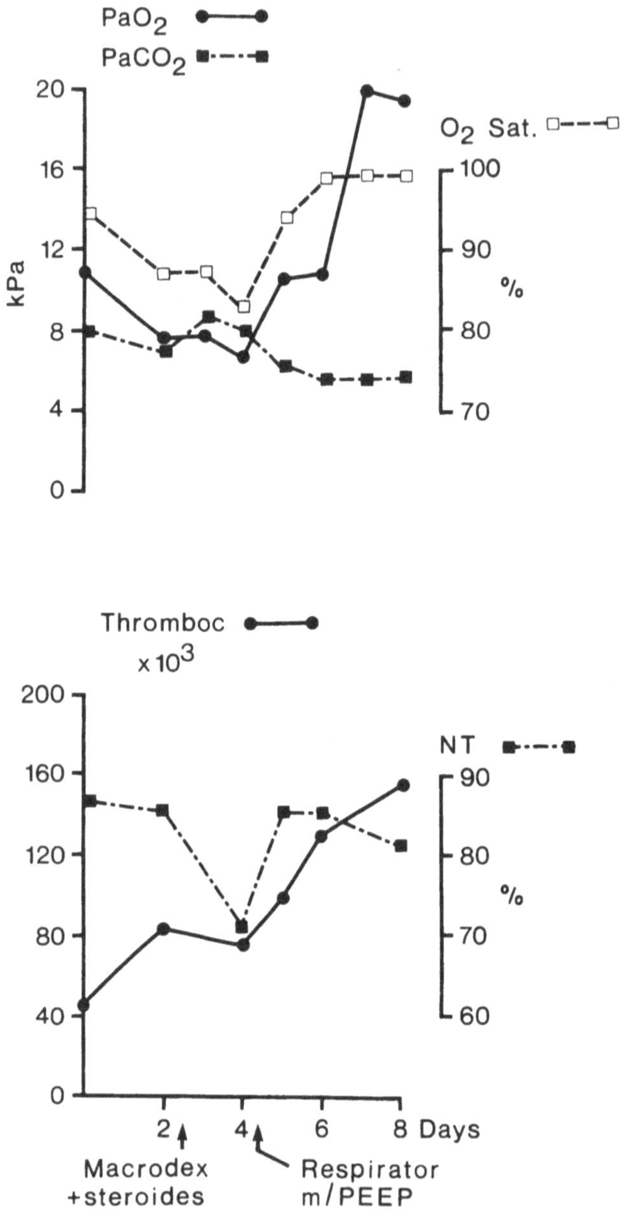


Figure 3

Changes in arterial $O_2$ tension, $CO_2$ tension, $O_2$ saturation, platelets and Normotest values in a patient (Case 1) with posttraumatic lung insufficiency.

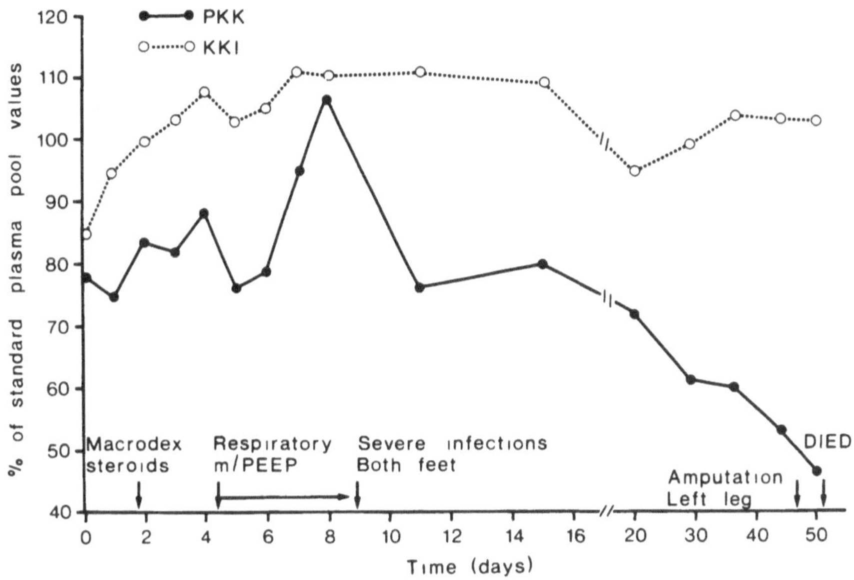


Figure 4

Changes in plasma prekallikrein and functional plasma kallikrein inhibitors in a patient with posttraumatic lung insufficiency (Case 1).

rupture was sutured and an osteotraction of the right leg was established. On the second day after admission, she developed respiratory problems with reduced arterial $0_2$-tension (5, 9 kPa) and thrombocytopenia. Respirator treatment was not instituted. Gradually the patients condition improved, and after 14 days osteo-synthesis with nailing of the tibia fracture was performed. The postoperative course passed without complications, and she left the hospital in good condition after 33 days.

In this patient also reduced PKK values were found during the first week after injury (fig. 5). Thereafter PKK values were normalized and found unchanged for the rest of the observation period. Functional kallikrein inhibition was normal for the whole observation period (fig. 5).

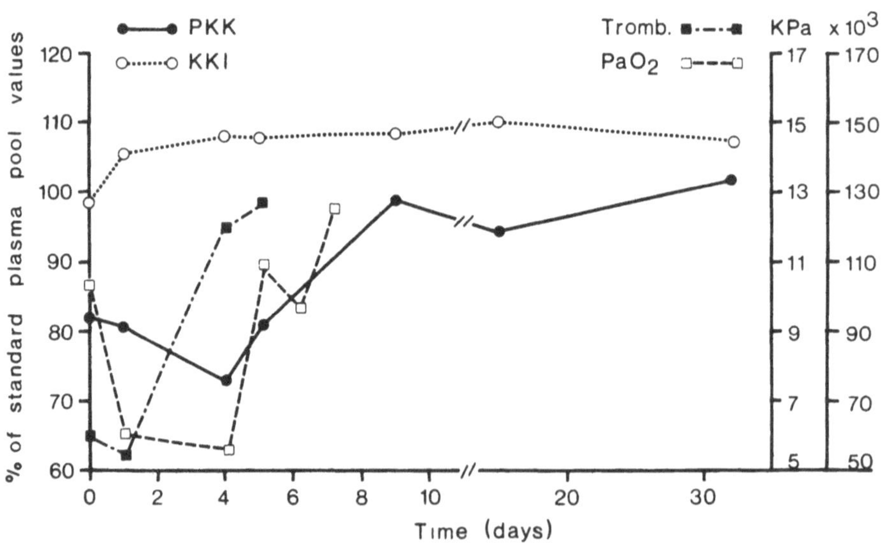


Figure 5

Changes in arterial $0_2$ tension, platelets and components of the plasma kallikrein-kinin system in a multitraumatized patient (Case 2) surviving posttraumatic respiratory distress.

<u>The Proenzyme functional inhibition index</u>

The plasma kallikrein kinin system is only one of the plasma protease systems which becomes activated in the traumatized patient. It is well documented that pronounced changes occur in the coagulation and fibrinolytic systems in this condition (10,11,13,24,29,31,36). From the information obtained by the changes seen for one or a few of the components of the plasma protease systems, it can be difficult to evaluate severity of the disease and closely monitor the patient.

This was the basis for development of the Proenzym functional inhibition index, PFI-index, (1). The PFI-index is calculated from chromogenic peptide substrate assays and is defined as the sum of deviation from the normal plasma pool values for

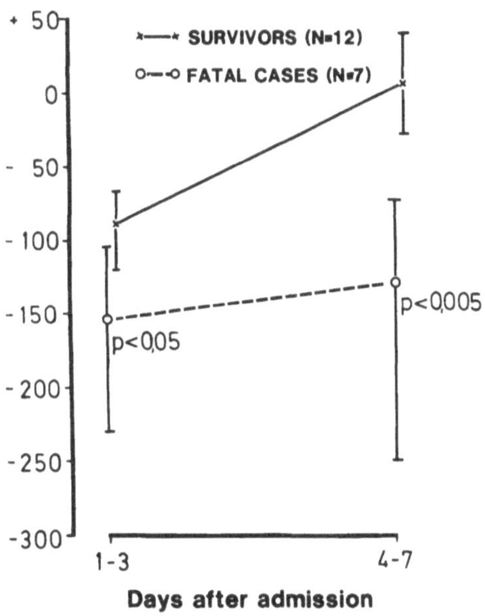


Figure 6

Proenzyme functional inhibition index values in 19 patients with multiple trauma. (Medium values, 25 and 75 percentiles, from (1).

the proenzyme and functional inhibition values for the coagulation, fibrinolytic and kallikrein-kinin systems (1). Increased values are counted as positive, whereas reductions compared with normal plasma pool values are recognized as negative.

In a recent study (1) PFI index values were found strongly negative in 19 patients with multiple trauma during the first three days after injury. The index values were significantly more negative in fatal cases than in survivors (fig. 6).

Index values were maintained strongly negative in fatal cases during the observation period, whereas values were normalized during the first week after the injury in survivors (fig. 6).

## DISCUSSION

The present paper summarizes changes found in the plasma kallikrein-kinin system during experimental posttraumatic shock and in patients with multiple trauma.

In both conditions evidence for activation of this protease system was found, demonstrated by reduced proenzyme values and functional inhibition activities and formation of plasma kallikrein-$\alpha_2$-macroglobulin complexes. The studies also demonstrate activation of other plasma protease systems after trauma (4,3).

Of particular interest were the observations that the reductions for several of the parameters studied were more pronounced in fatal cases than in survivors. These findings underline that the plasma protease systems are of great importance for maintaining homeostasis in the body.

Furthermore the present paper demonstrate that by means of the PFI-index the patients conditions as to severity and effect of treatment can be evaluated during early stages of the disease.

This information can be obtained by means of chromogenic peptide substrate assays which when automated are very suitable for use in intensive care medicine.

Another aspect of disclosing disturbances of the plasma protease systems in this state is that it establishes a basis for therapy.
Concentrates of plasma protease inhibitors regulating the activity in the coagulation (35,12) complement and kallikrein-kinin systems (Philapitsch 1983, personal communication) are now available. Furthermore activated plasma proteases as well as activators can be removed by means of plasmapheresis (McConn 1982, personal communication). Both these aspects of therapy can be closely monitored by means of chromogenic peptide substrate assays.

A majority of the fatal cases studied developed septicemia (1,3). The pronounced changes of the plasma protease systems seen in these patients is in accordance with recent studies on septicemia by our group (5,6,19,37,38,39), and others (15,18,22,25,42), and confirm that severe infection is a major threat to the traumatized patient.

## SUMMARY

The present paper summarizes recent studies by our group on the plasma kallikrein-kinin system in experimental post-traumatic shock and in patients with multiple trauma.

In both states extensive activation of this protease system was found. It is underlined that changes also occurs in several other protease systems as the coagulation and fibrinolytic systems following trauma.

In the multitraumatized patients significantly more pronounced reductions were found for several of the proteins studied in the fatal cases than in the survivors.

It is underlined that the changes can be closely monitored by chromogenic peptide substrate assays which are very suitable for intensive care medicine.

These assays are the basis for the application of a newly developed parament, the Proenzyme functional inhibition index. By means of this parameter the patients at high risks can be identified at an early stage after trauma.

ACKNOWLEDGEMENTS

The present studies have been financially supported by the Norwegian Research Council for Science and the Humanities and the Laerdal Foundation for Acute Medicine.

REFERENCES

1. Aasen A O. The proenzyme functional inhibition index. A new parameter for evaluation of the severely injured and septic patient. Act Chir Scand. In press.

2. Aasen A O, Kierulf P, Strømme J H. Methodological considerations on Chromogenic Peptide Substrate assays and application on automated analysers. Acta Chir Scand Suppl 1982; 509, pp. 17-23.

3. Aasen A O, Kierulf P, Vaage J, Godal H C, Aune S. Determination of components of the plasma proteolytic enzyme systems gives information of prognostic value in patients with multiple trauma. Adv Exp Med Biol 1983; 156 B, 1037.

4. Aasen A O, Saugstad O D, Lium B, Guldvog I, Lyngaas K, Larsbraaten M, Amundsen E. Plasma antiplasmin activities in experimental lung insufficiency. Acta Chir Scand 1980; 499, 113.

5. Aasen A L, Smith-Erichsen N, Amundsen E. Plasma kallikreinkinin system in septicemia. Arch Surg 1983; 118(3), 343.

6. Aasen A O, Smith-Erichsen N, Gallimore M J, Amundsen E. Studies on components of the plasma kallikreinaekinin system in plasma samples from normal individuals and patients with septic shock, In: "Advances in Shock Research" vol. 4, pp. 1, W. Schumer, J.J. Spitzer and B.E. Marshall, ed. Alan R. Liss, Inc. New York, 1980.

7. Amundsen E, Gallimore M J, Aasen A O, Larsbraaten M, Lyngaas K. Activation of human plasma prekallikrein: Influence av activators, activation and temperature and inhibitors. Thromb Res 1978; 13, 625.

8. Amundsen E, Svendsen L, Vennerød A M, Laake K. Determination of plasma kallikrein with a new chromogenic tripeptide derivative. In "chemistry and biology of the kallikrein-kinin system in health and disease". Proceedings No. 27, Washington DC, US Government Printing Office; 1977, pp. 215-220.

9. Bergström K, Blombäck M. Determination of Plasma Prothrombin with a Reaction Rate Analyzer Using a Synthetic Substrate. Thromb Res 1974; 4, 719.

10. Blaisdell F W, Lewis F R jr. Respiratory distress syndrome of shock and trauma. Philadelphia - London - Toronto, W.B. Saunders Co., 1977.

11. Blaisdell F W, Schlobohm M. The respiratory distress syndrome. A review, Surgery 1973; 74, 251.

12. Blauhot B, Necek, Vinazzer H, Bergman H. Substitution therapy with an antithrombin III concentrate in shock and DIC. Thromb Res 1982; 27, 271.

13. Bone R C, Francis P B, Pierce A K. Intravascular coagulation associated with the adult respiratory distress syndrome. Am J Med 1976; 61, 585.

14. Büller H R, Bowerk C, ten Cate J, Roos J, Kahlé L H, ten Cate J W. Postoperative hemostatic profile in relation to gramnegative septicemia. Critical Care Med; 1982, 10, 311.

15. ten Cate J W. Antithrombin-III: Clinical significance. Acta Chir Scand Suppl 1982: 509, pp. 101.

16. Cochrane C G, Griffin J H. Molecular Assembly in the contact phase of the Hageman Factor system. Am J Med 1979, 67, 657.

17. Colman R W. Formation of human plasma kinin. New Engl Med 1974; 5, 509.

18. Fritz H. Proteinase inhibitors in severe inflammatory process (septic shock and experimental endotoxaemia): biochemical, pathophysiological and therapeutic aspects. In: Chiba Foundation Symposium 75. Protein degradation in health and disease. 1980; pp. 351. Excerpta Medica.

19. Gallimore M J, Aasen A O, Smith-Erichsen N, Larsbraaten M, Lyngaas K, Amundsen E. Plasminogen concentrations and functional activities and concentrations of plasmin inhibitors in plasma samples from normal subjects and patients with septic shock. Throm Res 1980; 18, 601.

20. Harpel P C. Human plasma alpha$_2$ macroglobulin. An inhibitor of plasma kallikrein. J Exp Med 1970; 132, 329.

21. Heideman M, Kaijser B, Gelin L-E. Complement activation by homogenized muscle tissue. J Surg Res 1978; 25, 518.

22. Kalter E S, Timmermans A, Bouma B N. The kinin generating system during sepsis and bacterial shock. Agents and Actions Suppl 1982; 9, pp. 638.

23. Lium B, Saugstad O D, Aasen A O, Guldvog I, Nordstoga K, Amundsen E. Experimental Post-traumatic lung insufficiency in dogs. Acta vet Scand 1982; 23, 118.

24. Malik A B, van der Zee H. Mechanism of pulmonary Edema Induced by Microembolization in Digs. Circ Res 1978; 42, 72.

25. McConn R, Wasserman F, Haberland G. The Kallikreinkinin System in the Acutely Ill: Canges in Plasma Kininogen in Acutely Ill Patients and the Effiency of Pulmonary Clearance of Bradykinins. In: Role of Chemical Mediators in the Pathophysiology of Acute Illness and Injury. Raven Press, New York 1982; pp. 111.

26. Porcelli P, Foster W M, Bergofsky E H, Bicker A, Kaur R, Demeny M, Reich T. Pulmonary circulatory changes in pathogenesis of shock lung. Am J Med Sci 1974; 268, 250.

27. Ratnoff O D, Colopy J E. A familial hemorrhagic trait hemorrhagic trait associated with a deficiency of a clot-promoting fraction of plasma. J Clin Invest 1955;

28. Ratnoff O D, Pensky J, Ogston D, Naff G B. The inhibition of plasmin, plasma kallikrein, plasma permeability factor, and the Clr subcomponent of the first component of complement by serum C'l esterase inhibitor. J Exp Med 1969; 129, 315.

29. Risberg B. Fibrinolysis and trauma. Eur Surg Res 1978; 10, 373.

30. Saito H. The "Contact System" in Health and Disease. Adv in Inf Med 1980; 25, 217.

31. Saldeen T. The microembolism syndrome. Microvasc Res 1976; 11, 227.

32. Saugstad O D, Aasen A O, Guldvog I, Lium B, Larsbraaten M, Lyngaas K, Amundsen E. Activation of the kallikrein-kinin system during experimental lung insufficiency in dogs. Acta Chir Scand 1980; 499, 123.

33. Saugstad O D, Aasen A O, Guldvog I, Lium B, Lyngaas K, Amundsen E. Changes of components of the plasma kallikreinaekinin system during experimental lung insufficiency in dogs. Acta Chir Scand Suppl 1982; 509, 61.

34. Schapira M, Schott C F, Colamn R W. Contribution of plasma protease inhibitors to the inactivation of kallikrein in plasma. J Clin Invest 1982; 69, 462.

35. Schipper H G, Kahle L H, Jenkins C S P, ten Cate J W. Anti-thrombin III transfusion in disseminated intravascular coagulation. Lancet 1978; II, 854.

36. Seyfer A E, Seaber A V, Dombrose F A, Urbaniak J R. Coagulation changes in elective surgery and trauma. Ann Surg 1981; 193, 210.

37. Smith-Erichsen N, Aasen A O, Amundsen E. The functional inhibition of plasma kallikrein. A critical factor in septic shock. Adv Med Biol 1983; 156B, pp 927.

38. Smith-Erichsen N, Aasen A O, Amundsen E. Treatment of sepsis in the surgical patient evaluated by means of chromogenic peptide substrate assays. Acta Chir Scand Suppl 1982; 509, pp. 33.

39. Smith-Erichsen N, Aasen A O, Gallimore M J, Amundsen E. Studies of components of the coagulation system in normal Individuals and septic Shock patients. Circ Shock 1982; 9, 491.

40. Svendsen L, Blombäck M, Olsson P. Synthetic chromogenic substrates for determination of trypsin, thrombin and thrombin-like enzymes. Thromb Res 1972; 1, 267.

41. Svendsen, L., Amundsen, E. Estimation of plasmin and brinase activities by means of a highly susceptible

synthetic chromogenic peptide substrate. IVth International Congress on Thrombosis and Haemostasis, Vienna, (Abstract), 1973.

42. Witte J, Jochum M, Scheerer R, Schramm W, Hochstrasser K, Fritz H. Disturbances of selected plasma proteins in hyperdynamic septic shock. Intensive Care Med 1982; B, 215.

# DISTRIBUTION PATTERNS OF MICROTHROMBI IN DISSEMINATED INTRAVASCULAR COAGULATION (DIC)

*Studies in Autopsy Cases and Experimental Animals*

KAYAKO SHIMAMURA, M.D., KUNIYUKI OKA, M.D., MASAKI NAKAZAWA, M.D. AND MIZU KOJIMA, M.D.

Department of Pathology, College of Medical Technology and Nursing, University of Tsukuba, Ibaraki, Clinical Affairs Section, National Institute of Radiological Sciences, Chiba, Department of Haematology, Institute of Clinical Medicine, University of Tsukuba, and Department of Pathology, Institute of Basic Medical Science, University of Psukuba, Japan

## INTRODUCTION

In disseminated intravascular coagulation (DIC), microthrombi are known to be formed in systemic organs. However, their distribution differs from case to case, and different papers have reported various incidences of microthrombi in each organ (4,11,15). The present study is to clarify the distribution patterns of microthrombi in DIC and to elucidate how they occour.

First, we shall discuss the distribution patterns of microthrombi in human autopsy cases of untreated DIC, and later, those of rabbits with experimental DIC.

## STUDY OF HUMAN AUTOPSY CASES OF DIC

We studied thirtyseven autopsy cases of untreated DIC, as shown in Table I. None had a clinical diagnosis of DIC before autopsy. However, precise histological observation of each case disclosed enough microthrombi to label them DIC. Cases with thrombosis in large blood vessels were not included in this study, because it was difficult to distinguish microthrombi in DIC from thromboembolism secondary to the large vessel thrombosis.

| | |
|---|---|
| Number of Cases | 37 |
| Male : Female | 24 : 13 |
| Average Age | 61.8 yrs. |
| | (31-83 yrs) |

Criteria for selecting cases

1. Presence of multiple microthrombi in various organs
2. Absence of thrombosis in large blood vessels
3. No treatment for DIC

Table I. Cases Examined.

| Location | No. of Cases | Incidence(%) |
|---|---|---|
| Lung | 37 | 100.0 |
| Liver | 35 | 94.6 |
| Kidney | 28 | 75.5 |
| Heart | 21 | 56.8 |
| Pancreas | 18 | 48.7 |
| Adrenals | 12 | 32.4 |
| GI tract | 7 | 18.9 |

Table II. Incidence of Microthrombi

Table II shows the incidence of microthrombi in various organs. The lung was always affected, the liver and kidney quite frequently, and less commonly the other organs such as the heart, pancreas, adrenal glands and GI tract. Regarding to the lung, it was practically impossible to distinguish microthrombi from thromboembolism or fibrin aggregates secondary to tumor embolism. Therefore, microthrombi in the lung seemed to have little diagnostic value. The incidence of microthrombi in the heart, pancreas, adrenal glands and GI tract almost paralled with that in the liver &/or kidney. From these findings, we could consider the incidence of microthrombi in the liver and kidney a good indicator of systemic distribution of microthrombi in DIC.

Based on this observation, we reexamined histological slides of each case with special reference to the numbers of microthrombi in the liver and kidney. In the liver, we counted the number of microthrombi per square centimeter of each section and in the kidney, we calculated the percentage of glomeruli with microthrombi. As shown in Fig. 1, four distribution patterns were distinguishable: hepatic, hepatorenal, renal and undetermined. The hepatic pattern was defined as that in which more than 20 microthrombi per square centimeter of liver section were present, but less than 20 % of glomeruli were microthrombosed. The hepatorenal pattern was characterized by

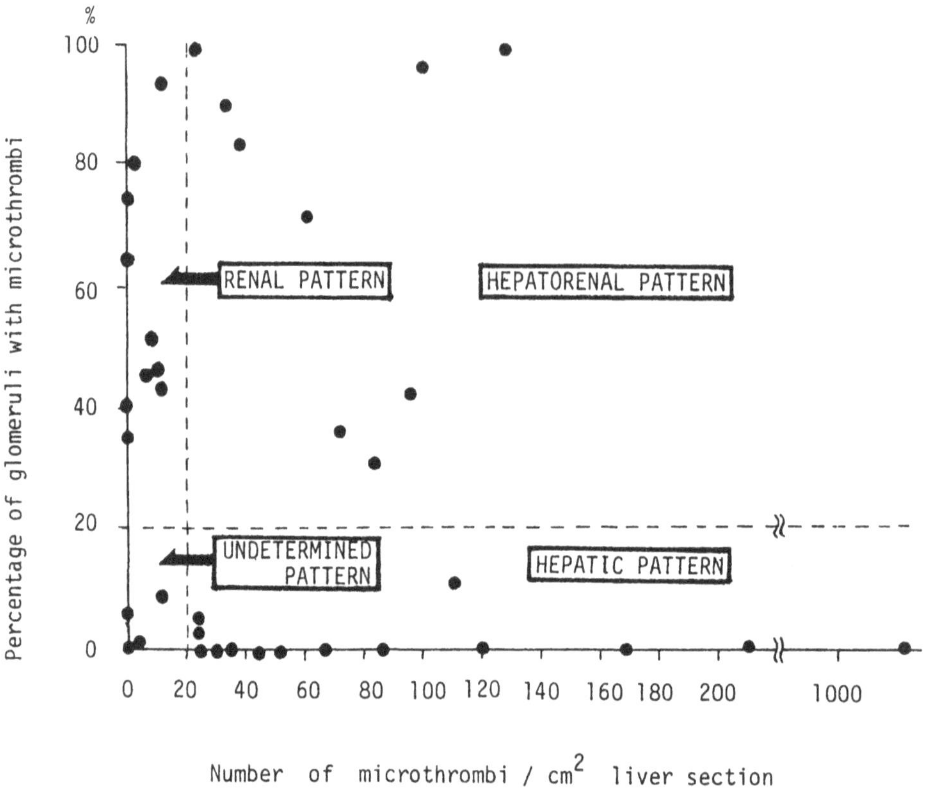


Figure 1

Relationship between numbers of microthrombi in liver and kidney in each case.

the presence of 20 or more microthrombi per square centimeter of liver section and microthrombosis in over 20 % of glomeruli. The renal pattern was the one in which more than 20 % of glomeruli were affected but less than 20 microthrombi were recognized in one square centimeter of liver section. Other cases with only a few microthrombi each were classified as the undetermined pattern. Characteristics of each pattern were summarized in Table III.

Hepatic pattern

Fourteen subjects (eleven men and three women) showed hepatic patterns. Their average age was 60.3 years (range, 31 to 83 years). Underlying disease included malignant tumours in 10 patients (three with gastric carcinoma; two pancreatic carci-

| Distribution Patterns (No.of Cases) | Incidence of Microthrombi Liver No/sq cm | Glomeruli % | Others | Incidence of Organizing Microthrombi | Thrombolysis | Renal Injury |
|---|---|---|---|---|---|---|
| Hepatic (14) | 145.5 | 1.4 | few | 28.6 | none | none |
| Hepatorenal (9) | 70.4 | 71.9 | a few | 4.5 | slight | slight |
| Renal (10) | 5.0 | 67.7 | a few | 50.0 | marked | marked |
| Undetermined (4) | 4.0 | 3.5 | few | 25.0 | - | none |

Table III. Characteristics of Four Distribution Patterns of Microthrombi

noma; one each with lung, kidney, and colon carcinoma; and two with leukemia), septicemia in two, severe burn in one and cranial trauma in one.

The average number of microthrombi in hepatic sinusoids was 145.4/sq cm, and the incidence of glomeruli with microthrombi was 1.4 %. A small number of microthrombi was also found in other organs; 18.7/sq cm in the lung, 1.9/sq cm in the adrenal gland, and 0.3/sq cm in the heart. The average number of organs with microthrombi was 3.6.

According to morphological criteria of the age of microthrombi, which the authors have reported before(6, 16a), 42,8 % of microthrombi in the various organs in these subjects were fresh, not being covered with endothelial cells. The incidence of aged organized microthrombi was 28.6 %. The duration of DIC was retrospectively estimated from the clinical data, and less than a 14-day duration was found in all subjects.

Kupffer's cells in these subjects adsorbed fibrin strands in the hepatic sinusoids or engulfed them into cytoplasm (Fig. 2). Therefore, it seemes that Kupffer's cells were active in clearing fibrin.

Hepatorenal pattern

The nine patients (three men and six women) in this group had

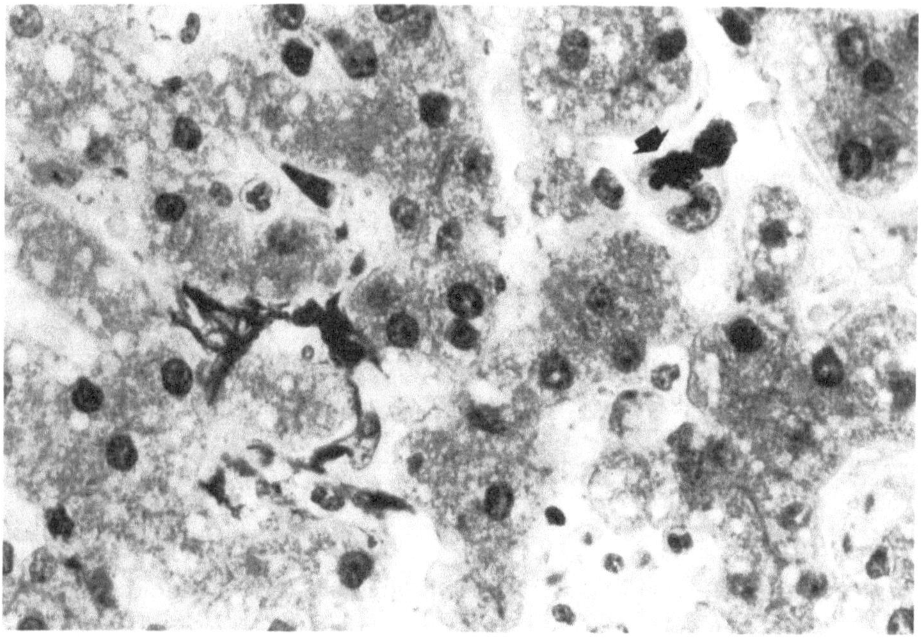

Figure 2

Microthrombi in the hepatic sinusoids in hepatic pattern of DIC. They attach to Kupffer's cells and some of them seem to be engulfed in the cytoplasm (arrow). (PTAH stain, original magnification x 400).

an average of 61 years (range, 52 to 73 years). Underlying diseases were malignant tumors in five patients (two of each with gastric and lung carcinoma, respectively, and one with esophageal carcinoma), two septicemia, and one each of encephalomalacia and postoperative ileus. The estimated duration of DIC varied from less than one week to more than three weeks.

The average number of microthrombi in the hepatic sinusoids was 70.4/sq cm, and 71.9 % of glomeruli contained microthrombi. Microthrombi were detected frequently in other organs as well; 23.4/sq cm in the lung, 7.5/sq cm in the adrenal gland, 1.3/sq cm in the pancreas, and 0.7/sq cm in the heart. An average of five organs had microthrombi. 44.5% of the microthrombi were organizing and therefore aged. Two patients were found to have renal tubular necrosis.

Kupffer's cells in these patients also showed adsorption or

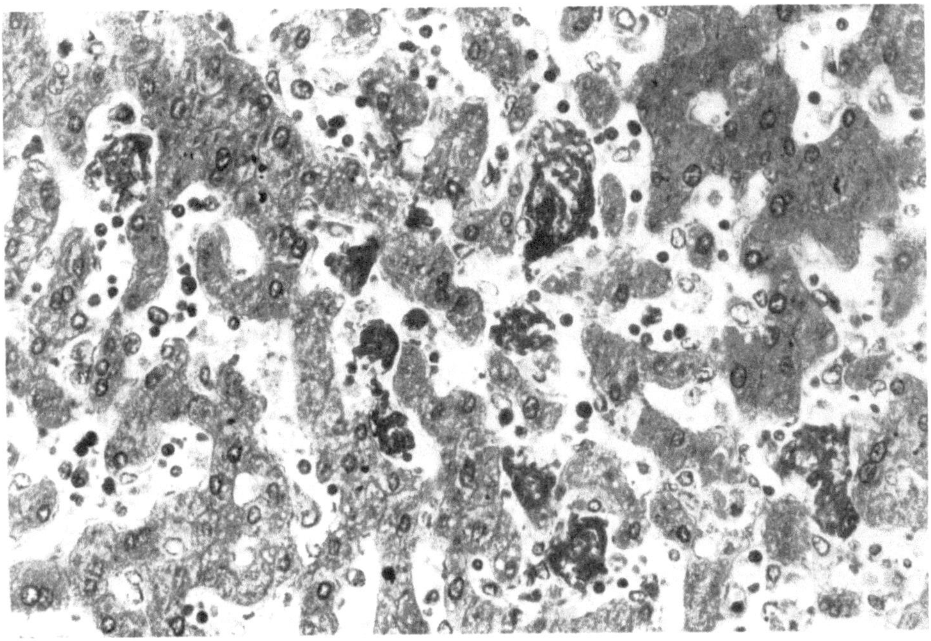

Figure 3

Microthrombi in the hepatic sinusoids in hepatorenal pattern of DIC. Many fibrin aggregates flocculate apart from Kupffer's cells. (HE stain, original magnification x 200).

engulfment of microthrombi as was seen in the hepatic pattern. Moreover, there were free fibrin aggregates in the hepatic sinusoids (Fig. 3), and polymorphonuclear leukocyte aggregates around the microthrombi. Based on these findings, it seemed that hepatorenal pattern cases were caused by the overproduction of fibrin beyond the clearing capacity of Kupffer's cells; in other words, the "spilling over"(1) of fibrin or related substances from the liver to the peripheral blood flow induced the formation of microthrombi in the various organs.

Renal pattern

In the ten subjects (eight men and two women) in this group, the average oage was 65.9 years (range, 50 to 76 years). Underlying diseases were malignant tumors in five cases (two gastric carcinoma, one lung, one pancreas, and one malignant lymphoma), septicemia in three, and bronchopneumonia in one and hemorrhagic ileitis in one. The estimated duration of DIC varied from four days to one month.

An average of 67.7 % of glomeruli had microthrombi, and the average number of them in the hepatic sinusoids was 5/sq cm. A small number of microthrombi was also found in other organs; 25.8/sq cm in the lung, 1.7/sq cm in the adrenal gland, and 0.5/sq cm in the heart. An average of 4.5 organs were involved.

Bilaterial cortical necrosis and focal tubular necrosis were observed in three out of ten cases. Microthrombi in the glomeruli showed various stages of thrombolysis (Fig. 4). Generally, the percentage of organized microthrombi in the various organs was 50 %, and thrombolysis was often observed. These data suggest that renal pattern cases had a longer duration of DIC than those of the hepatic and hepatorenal patterns.

According to these findings, we came to the hypothesis that the generation of microthrombi starts with the hepatic pattern at the beginning, which is followed by the hepatorenal pattern, and then by the renal pattern. These patterns of distribution and no relationship with the underlying diseases or the extent of tissue injury of the liver and kidney.

Undetermined pattern

Four patients (two men and two women) belonged to this group, whose average age was 60 years (range, 42 to 71 years). The underlying diseases were malignant tumor in three patients (two esophageal carcinomas and one multiple myeloma) and cor pulmonale due to pulmonary silicosis in one. An average of 4.1 organs had microthrombi. Although the average number of microthrombi in the hepatic sinusoids was 4/sq cm, there were no microthrombi in the hepatic sinusoids in two of four cases. On the average, microthrombi were found in 3.5 % of all glomeruli. They numbered 12.3/sq cm in the lung and 0.4/sq cm in the heart. They were considered either a prehepatic or postrenal pattern.

## STUDY OF EXPERIMENTAL ANIMALS WITH DIC

In order to substantiate the hypothesis that distribution patterns of microthrombi show a chronological aspect of tran-

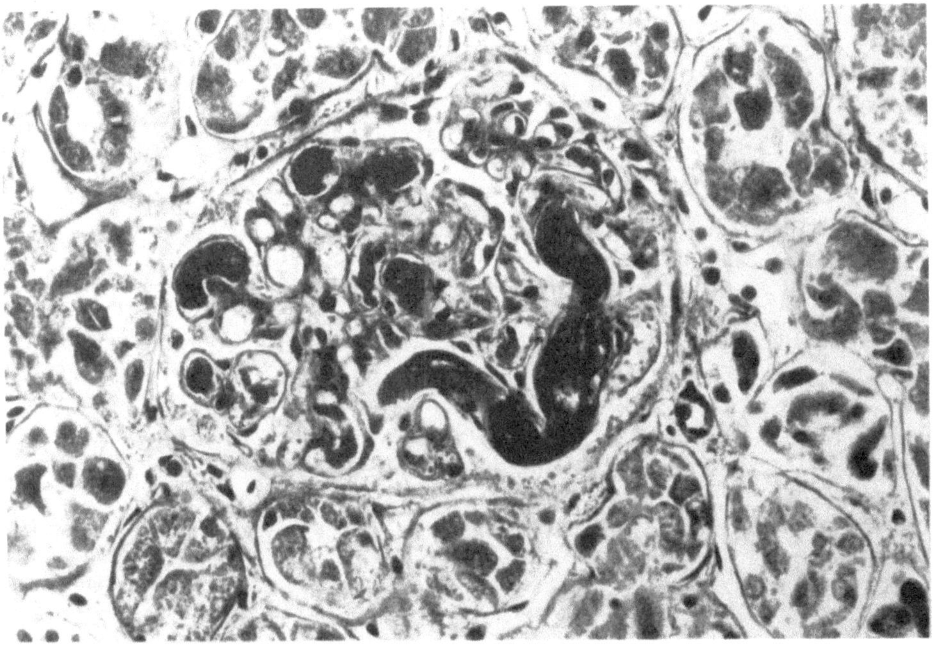

Figure 4

Process of thrombolysis in a renal glomerulus in renal pattern of DIC. Some microthrombi completely obstruct the capillary loops, while others are reduced in size and are scattered inside the loops. Finally, only empty loops with thickened wall are left, where the microthrombi were completely lysed. (picro-Mallory stain, original magnification x 200 ).

sition from hepatic to hepatorenal and then to renal, the distribution patterns of microthrombi during the course of generalized Shwartzman phenomenon were investigated (5,7,10). This phenomenon is a highly developed form of DIC induced by two injections of endotoxin, and it is suitable as an experimental model of human DIC.

Male albino rabbits weighing 2 to 3 kg received two intravenous injections of endotoxin (Difco, USA) into ear veins in a dose of 200 µg/kg body weight with an interval of 24 hours. As shown in Fig. 5, 30 minutes after the second injection, microthrombi first appeared in the hepatic sinusoids, and after the course of three to six hours, they disseminated systemically and then gradually disappeared.

The disappearance of microthrombi also first took place in the

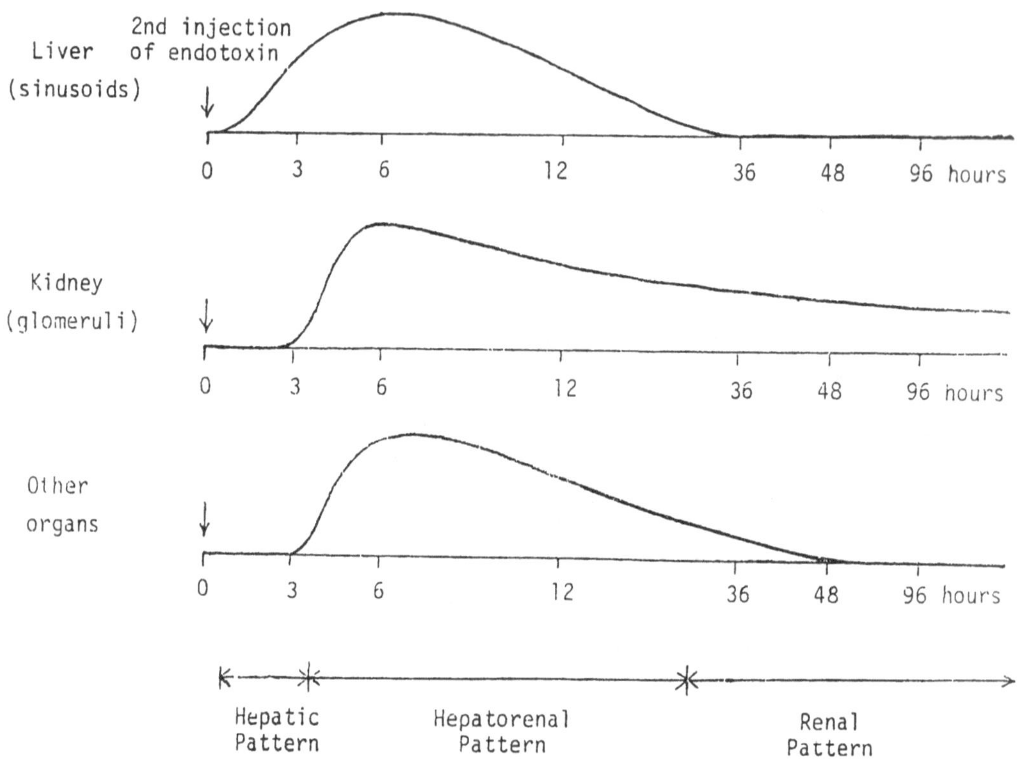


Figure 5

Distribution of microthrombi in generalized Shwartsman phenomenon

hepatic sinusoids, and microthrombi in the kidney remained longer. In other words, this model using experimental animals showed the same course of DIC as was observed in the human autopsy cases. Under the electron microscope, during the early phase of this phenomenon, microthrombi in the hepatic sinusoids were adhered to Kupffer's cells or they seemed engulfed in the cytoplasm, as if they were phagocytised. There have been controversial observations regarding to the phagocytosis of fibrin aggregates by Kupffer's cells (2,3,8,9,14,17). In the present study, most of the fibrin-containing phagosome-like structures opened into the sinuosidal space and furthermore, they showed negative acid phophatase activity (Fig. 6). Therefore, we can assume that phagosome-like structures were caused by complicated invagination of plasma membrane and that they are

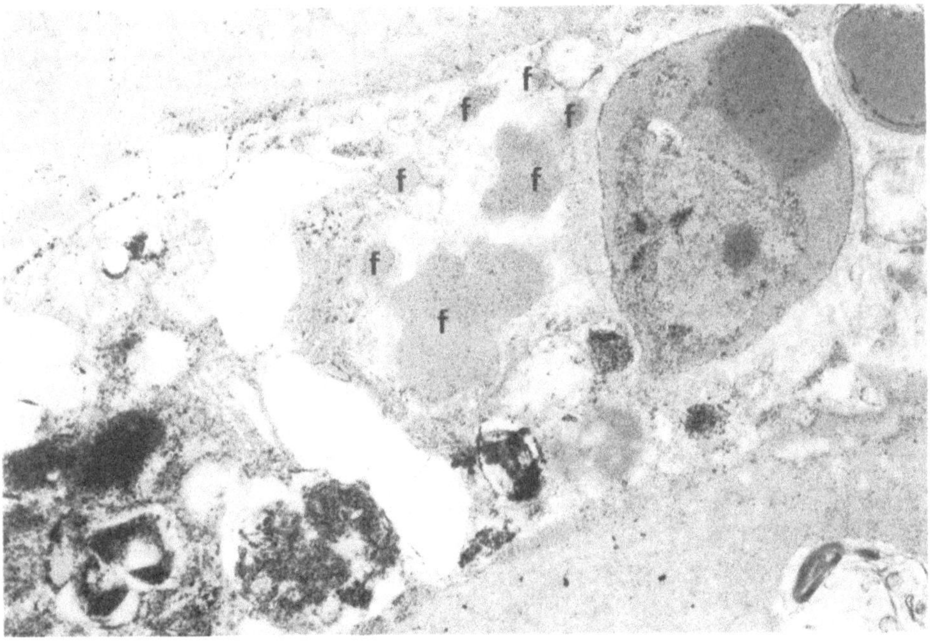


Figure 6

Kupffer's cell of a rabbit 8 hours after second injection of endotoxin. Fibrin strands ( f ) seem to be engulfted into the cytoplasm, but phagosome-like structures containing fibrin strands are negative for acid phosphatase activity. Electron microscopical acid phosphatase staining, original magnification x 5000 ).

not profile of phagocytosis. Our data coincide with those of Emeis et al (3) who reported that Kupffer's cells adsorbed fibrin on their surface but did not phagocytise them. Then a question arose as to the process of fibrin clearing activity of Kupffer's cells. To answer this question, an electron microscopical study on the fibrin clearing activity of Kupffer's cells was performed using thrombin-infused rabbits (7,12). The reason why we did not use endotoxin injected rabbits was that endotoxin has a tendency to damage Kupffer's cells.

A 10 U/ml thrombin solution was infused into the portal vein of rabbits at a rate of 0.33 ml/min using perista minipump. After the infusion of 50 U, fibrin began to adhere selectively to the surface of Kupffer's cells as shown in the scheme. 200 U of thrombin caused the increase of fibrin on the surface of Kupffer's cells and the invagination of plasma membrane (Fig. 7). Sometimes complicated invagination of plasma membrane formed labyrinth-like structures. The distance between fibrin and plasma membrane of Kupffer's cells ranged from

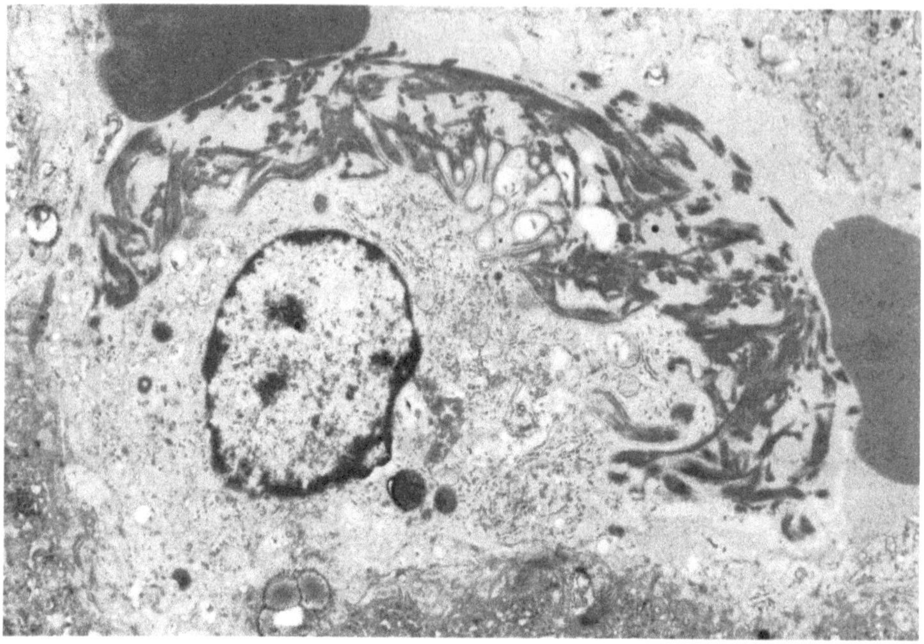

Figure 7

Kupffer's cell of a rabbit after infusion of 200 U of thrombin. Thick fibrin bundles envelop the cell surface, and invagination of plasma membrane is prominent, (original magnification x 2000)

50 to 70 nm, which corresponded to the width of the cell coat (13). When the infusion of thrombin was stopped at this point, many bristle coated vesicles appeared around the invaginated portions of plasma membrane (Fig. 8), which suggests that fibrin is cleared by pinocytosis. Namely, fibrin seems to be lysed, taken up into bristle coated vesicles by pinocytosis then digested by Kupffer's cells.

With over 200 units of thrombin infused, free fibrin aggregates were found in the hepatic sinusoids as well as the microthrombi adhered to Kupffer's cells. Light microscopically, microthrombi were detected not only in the hepatic sinusoids but also in 35 % of renal glomeruli. This suggests that the clearing activity of Kupffer's cells is limited to the amount of fibrin formed at this stage.

From these experiments using endotoxin and thrombin, we can assume that when fibrin generation exceeds the maximum clear-

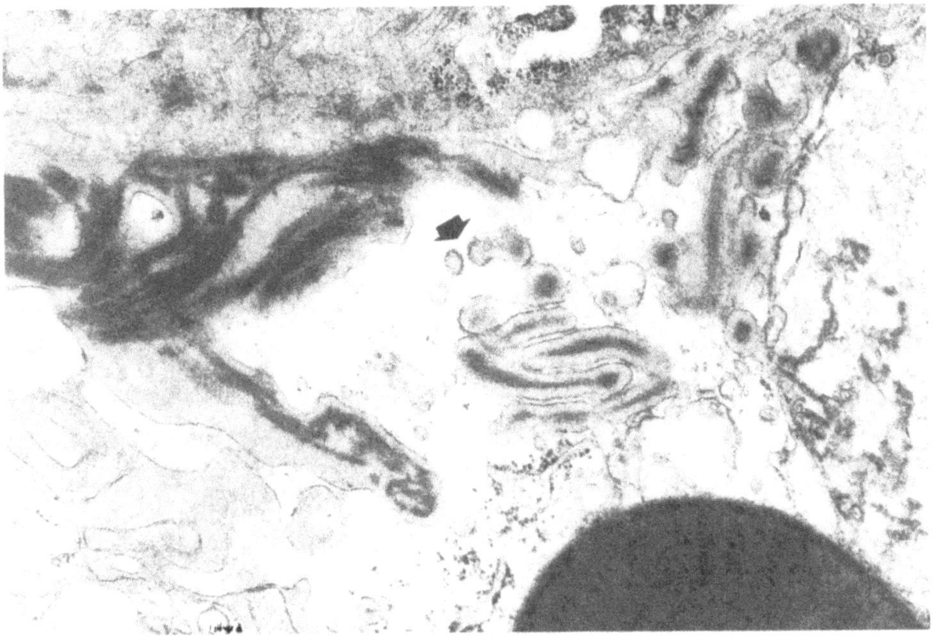

Figure 8

Kupffer's cell of a rabbit 30 minutes after stopping infusion of 200 U of thrombin. Many bristle coated vesicles are seen in the vicinity of invaginated plasma membrane ( arrow ), (original magnification x 2000 )

ing capacity of Kupffer's cells, microthrombi are disseminated in systemic organs. That is, the "spilling over" of fibrin or substances causing intravascular coagulation such as endotoxin or thrombin from the liver to systemic circulation can be considered to trigger disseminated intravascular coagulation.

Further studies are warranted to clarify the mechanism of fibrin clearing activity of Kupffer's cells.

## SUMMARY

Distribution patterns of microthrombi in disseminated intravascular coagulation (DIC) were morphologically studied using 37 autopsy cases of untreated DIC and rabbit with generalized Shwartzman phenomenon as well as thrombin-infused rabbits. According to the organs predominantly involved, four patterns were distinguished : hepatic, hepatorenal, renal and undeter-

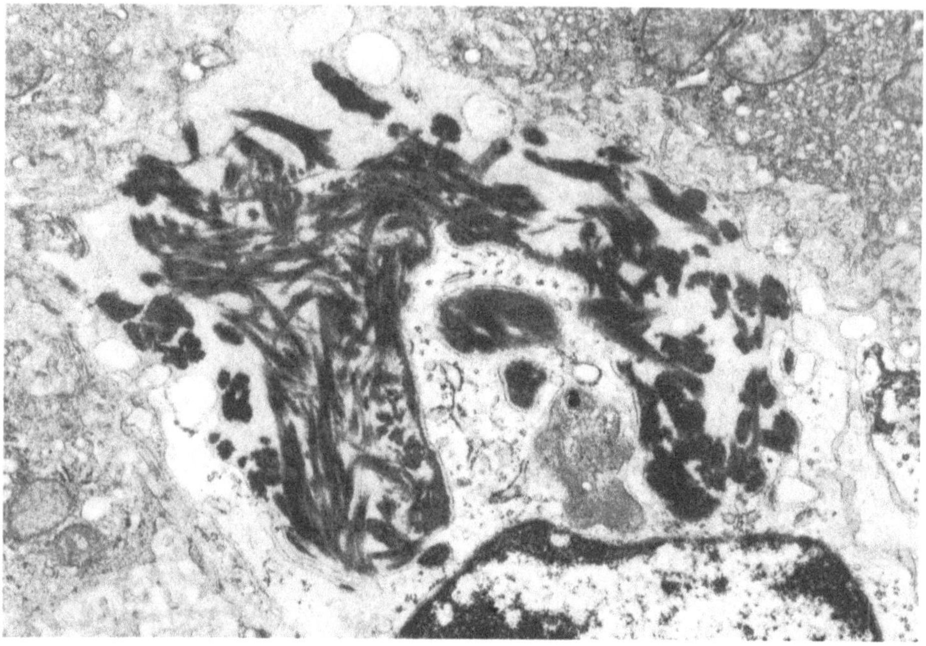

Figure 9

Kupffer's cell of a rabbit after infusion of 400 U of thrombin. Fibrin strands surrounding Kupffer's cell are being detached from Kupffer's cell ( original magnification x 5000 )

mined. The results suggest that in the course of DIC, the hepatic pattern appears first, followed by the hepatorenal pattern, and then renal pattern. The undetermined pattern is considered to correspond to either prehepatic or postrenal pattern. Dissemination of microthrombi in systemic organs seems to be induced when fibrin generation exceeds the maximum clearing capacity of Kupffer cells.

## ACKNOWLEDGEMENT

This study was supported by the Ministry of Education, Culture and Science of Japan and the research grant for DIC from the Ministry of Health and Welfare of Japan.

We wish to thank Dr. H. Wakasa, Fukushima Medical College, Fukushima, Japan and Dr. H. Hakozaki, Fukushima Rosai Hospital, Fukushima, Japan, for kindly giving us a chance to review their DIC cases.

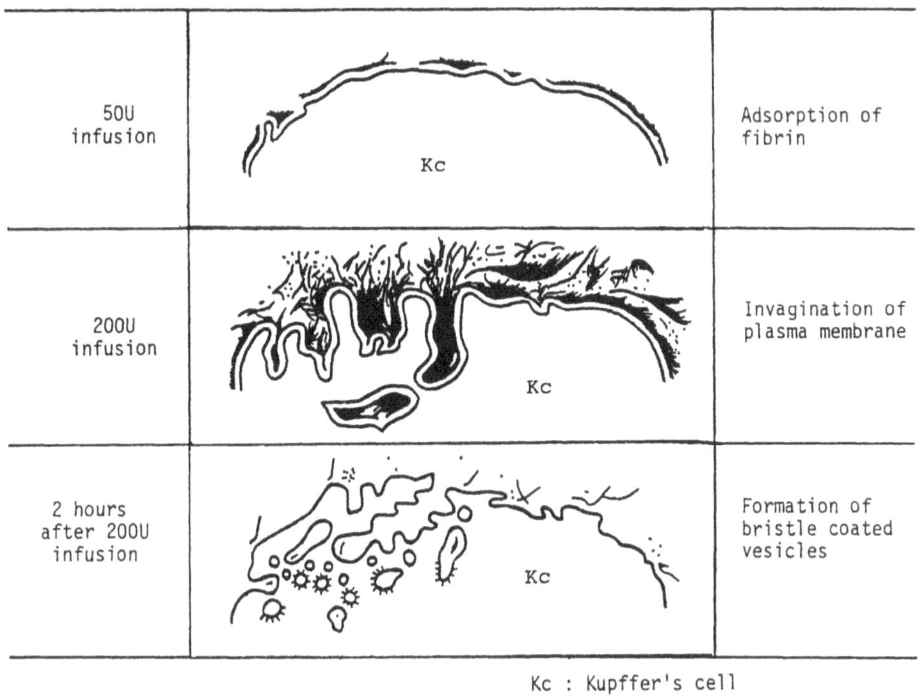


Figure 10

Fibrin clearance by Kupffer's cell

## REFERENCES

1. Bradfield JWB. Can we measure Kupffer cell function in man? In: The Reticuloendothelial System and the Pathogenesis of Liver Disease (Liehr H and Grün M eds.), Elsevier, North-Holland Biochemical Press, 1980; 309-316.

2. Emeis JJ, Brederoo P. The cell coat of macrophage. In: the Reticuloendothelial system (Friedman H, Escobar M and Reichard SM eds.) Morphology (edited by Carr I and Daems WT), Plenum Press, New York-London, 1980; 129-159.

3. Emeis JJ, Lindeman J. Rat liver macrophages will not phagecytose fibrin during disseminated intravascular coagulation. Haemostasis 1976; 5:193-210.

4. Kim HS, Suzuki M, Lie JT et al. Clinically unsuspected disseminated intravascular coagulation: An autopsy survey. Am J Clin Path, 1976; 66:31-39.

5. Kojima M, Shimamura K, Kanari T. Endotoxin and DIC. In: DIC and Allied Condition (Aoki N, Matsuda T, Mori W, Tamakuma M eds.), Ishiyaku Shuppan, 1980; 66-72.

6. Kojima M, Shimamura K, Mori N, Oka K, Nakazawa M. A histological study on microthrombi in autopsy cases of DIC. In: Disseminated Intravascular Coagulation (Abe T and Yamanaka M eds,), University of Tokyo Press, 1983; 95-106.

7. Kojima M, Shimamura K, Nakazawa M, Oka K. Kupffer cell and disseminated intravascular coagulation. Rec Adv RES (in press).

8. Lee L, McCluskey RT. Immunohistochemical demonstration of the reticuloendothelial clearance of circulating fibrin aggregates. J Exp Med, 1962; 116:611-618.

9. Margaretten W, Zunker HO, McKay DJ. Production of the generalized Scwartzman reaction in pregnant rats by intravenous infusion of thrombin. Lab Invest, 1964; 13:552-559.

10. Nakazawa M, Shimamura K, Oka K, Kojima M. Role of Kupffer cells in disseminated intravascular coagulation. Morphologic study on endotoxin injected rabbits. J RES (submitted)

11. Nozicka Z, Votel V. Histological picture of acute disseminated intravascular coagulation. Cesk Pathol, 1975; 11: 90-95.

12. Oka K, Shimamura K, Nakazawa M, Kojima M. Role of Kupffer cells in disseminated intravascular coagulation. Morphologic study on thrombin-infused rabbits. Arch Pathol Lab Med (in press).

13. Pfeifer U. Über Endocytose in Kupfferschen Sternzellen nach Parenchymschädingung durch 3/4 Teilkepatektomie. Virchows Arch B, 1970; 6:263-280.

14. Prose PH, Lee L, Balk SD. Electron microscopic study of the phagocytic fibrin-clearing mechanism. Am J Pathol, 1965; 47:403-417.

15 Robboy SJ, Colman RW, Minna JD. Pathology of disseminated intravascular coagulation: Analysis of 26 cases. Hum Pathol, 1972. 3:327-343.

16a. Shimamura K, Kojima M. Removal of fibrin thrombi in disseminated intravascular coagulation (DIC). Morphological studies. Arch Pathol Lab Med, 1981; 105: 659-663.

16b. Shimamura K, Oka K, Nakazawa M, Kojima M. Distribution patterns of microthrombi in disseminated intravascular coagulation (DIC). Arch Pathol Lab Med (in press).

17. Still WJS, Scott GBD. An electorn microscopic study of the endothelial changes and the nature of "Fibrinoid" produced in the generalized Shwartzman reaction. Exp Mol Pathol, 1966; 5:118-124.

# BLOOD COAGULATION AND RELATED SYSTEMS IN THE PATHOGENESIS OF ACUTE RESPIRATORY DISTRESS

TOM SALDEEN, M.D., Ph.D.

Department of Forensic Medicine,
University of Uppsala
Uppsala, Sweden

The adult respiratory distress syndrome (ARDS) continues to be a major cause of morbidity and mortality after trauma and sepsis. It is estimated that there are 150 000 cases in the United States each year (21),the mortality being 40-50 percent (28, 48). Despite intensive research, the survival rates for patients with ARDS have remained unchanged during the last 15 years. Most of the cases of acute respiratory distress after trauma have well-known causes, such as pulmonary edema due to left heart failure or fluid overload, pneumonia, aspiration, postoperative atelectasis, blunt chest trauma, macrothromboembolism, and, especially, septicemia. About 10 percent are idiopathic cases and it is these with which this paper will deal.

One hundred autopsies of patients whose deaths were caused by acute idiopathic respiratory distress after trauma have been performed in our department during the last 18 years, these constituting 0.7 percent of our autopsy cases. What is most interesting in these cases is the presence of fibrin in small pulmonary arterial branches and capillaries (54). Electron microscopy of biopsy specimens from the lungs also shows deposition of fibrin between and outside the endothelial cells, as the most characteristic feature (45). Moreover, in post-traumatic patients who are given labelled fibrinogen intravenously, a large increase in the radioactivity over the lungs is seen in those who develop respiratory insufficiency, but no such uptake is found in those patients at risk who do not develop pulmonary symptoms (12). This radioactivity increase, indicating fibrin deposition, is associated temporally with the onset of the respiratory insufficiency, suggesting a causal relationship between the trapping of fibrin and the pulmonary damage.

Concerning the mechanism underlying the trapping of fibrin in the lungs, there is evidence that in trauma cases the intravascular coagulation is induced by thromboplastin released from the injured area. Thus, there is a good correlation between thromboplastin activity in the pulmonary arterial blood and a decrease in $pO_2$ (46). In the patients with sepsis the intravascular coagulation may be induced by thromboplastin synthesized by monocytes as a result of stimulation by endotoxin, for example. Many observations indicate that the fibrin in the lungs is a consequence of microembolization from the venous circulation (7, 54).

The trapping of fibrin in the lungs after severe injury occurs in two different phases: an initial transient phase, and a secondary, more pronounced and more long-standing phase starting about two days after the trauma and with a maximum at 7 days. These two phases have been called the early microembolism syndrome and the delayed microembolism syndrome, respectively (Figs 1 and 2) (54).

In the early phase the microemboli cause an increase in the synthesis of thromboxane $A_2$, resulting in pulmonary vasoconstriction and bronchiolar constriction. Most of the thromboxane is probably released from pulmonary vessels as a consequence of damage induced by the microemboli and by certain products released during the degradation of fibrin. Thromboxane released from platelet and leukocyte aggregates may also contribute to the changes in blood and airway pressures.

Low molecular weight degradation products of fibrin induce release of thromboxane from the pulmonary vascular bed and an increase in pulmonary vascular resistance and bronchiolar constriction (1). Since their discovery in the mid- 1970s, thromboxane and prostacyclin have been found to have a strong vasoactive effects, thromboxane being a vasoconstrictor and prostacyclin a vasodilator. Prostacyclin is produced in the vessel wall. It has been assumed, on the other hand, that thromboxane is not present in the vessel wall, or only in amounts insignificant from a patho-physiological point of view. Recent evidence has shown, however, that damaged blood vessels have a high capacity to produce thromboxane (51). The thromboxane may be produced partly by leukocytes trapped on or in the vessel walls (52). It is thus probably that microemboli in the lung, by causing vascular damage and release of fibrin degradation products, induce production of thromboxane, with vasoconstriction or broncho-constriction as a result. Low molecular weight degradation products of fibrin will also release prostacyclin from peripheral vessels, leading to peripheral vasodilation (2). These products also release histamine in the lungs, which can result in pulmonary vasoconstriction and bronchoconstriction (54).

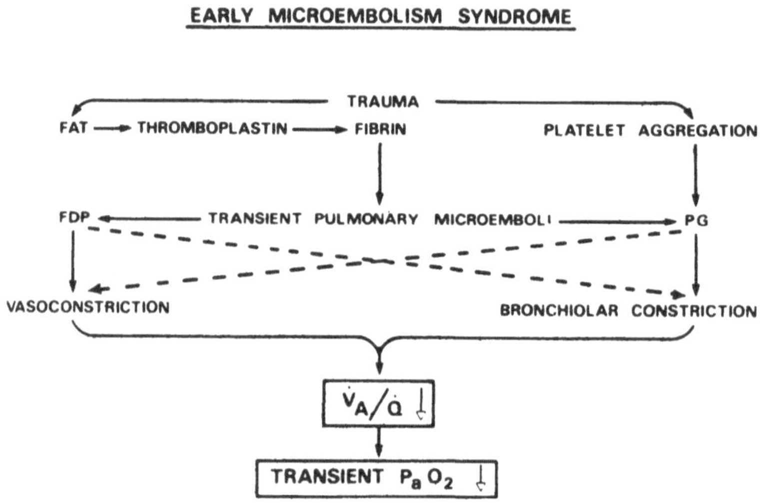


Figure 1.

Pathogenesis of the early microembolism syndrome. FDP = fibrin degradation products, PG = prostaglandins. $\dot{V}_A/\dot{Q}$ = ventilation-perfusion ratio. $P_aO_2$ = arterial oxygen tension.

The early form of the syndrome is often subclinical, with transient trapping of microemboli in the lungs, giving rise to a transient decrease in $pO_2$ and arterial blood pressure. Occasionally, however, the reaction can be very severe, with extreme vasoconstriction, severe hypotension with shock, and death, probably due to right heart failure. The signs of respiratory insufficiency in the delayed microembolism syndrome are a progressive decrease in $pO_2$ and in the ratio of arterial to alveolar $pO_2$, due to a decreased ventilation-perfusion ratio and a gradually developing right-left shunt (54). The most important finding from a pathological-anatomical point of view is the protein-rich edema. There is an increase in pulmonary vascular resistance which may be partly due to vascular compression caused by the edema.

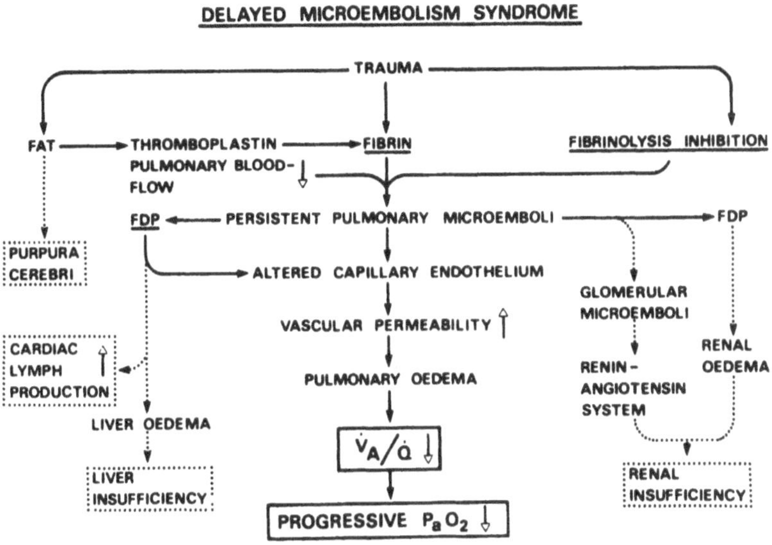


Figure 2.

Schematic diagram of the pathogenesis of the delayed microembolism syndrome. For abbreviations, see Fig. 1.

The presence of fibrin in the lungs of patients with the delayed microembolism syndrome points not only to intravascular coagulation but also to a disturbance of the fibrinolytic system. Normally the lungs can efficiently remove and degrade fibrin trapped in the pulmonary vessels (53).

A defect, namely a high concentration of fibrinolysis inhibitors in the blood, makes these patients less able to degrade the fibrin. One important inhibitor is $\alpha_2$-antiplasmin or the primary fibrinolysis inhibitor (PFI).

This inhibitor is produced in the liver (36). An increased amount of circulating free fatty acids is associated with an increase in this inhibitor in the blood (56). There are two forms of the protein in the blood, both of which react to the antibodies against the inhibitor. One of these forms has affinity for plasminogen and is a very efficient plasmin inhibitor - "primary fibrinolysis inhibitor: alpha". The other form has no affinity for plasminogen and is a much weaker inhibitor of plasmin. Only the alpha form is increased after trauma (3).

The results of a study of primary fibrinolysis inhibitor: alpha in patients with a risk of developing the delayed microembolism syndrome after multiple trauma are illustrated in Fig. 3. Patients in whom the syndrome subsequently developed showed an increased concentration of this inhibitor, in contrast to those in whom it did not develop (4). Both groups of patients had low platelet counts, and it is important to note that both intravascular coagulation and a large increase in primary fibrinolysis inhibitor: alpha are prerequisites for the the occurrence of this syndrome. Intravascular coagulation or inhibited fibrinolysis alone is not sufficient. Some authors have reported a correlation between a decrease in fibronectin in the blood and development of acute respiratory failure (49), but this was not confirmed in our study mentioned above.

Another inhibitor that is increased in patients with the delayed microembolism syndrome is the recently discovered fast acting inhibitor of tissue plasminogen activator (17, 38) (Fig. 4).

It thus seems that trapping of fibrin in the lungs with decreased elimination of fibrin due to an increase in inhibitors of fibrinolysis may be one pathogenetic factor in the microembolism syndrome. Different observations indicate that the fibrin contributes to the increased vascular permeability by a mechanism other than by causing mechanical blockage and that products of fibrin degradation released locally in the pulmonary tissue from persistent microemboli in the lungs may be involved. Some peptides produced by plasmin degradation of fibrin, namely a pentapeptide and an undecapeptide, which increase vascular permeability, have been isolated (6), and recently also some peptides produced by elastase degradation of fibrin, which have potent permeability-increasing effects (61, 63). Leukocytes and elastase are found in large amounts in the alveoli of patients with the delayed microembolism syndrome (37, 39, 44).

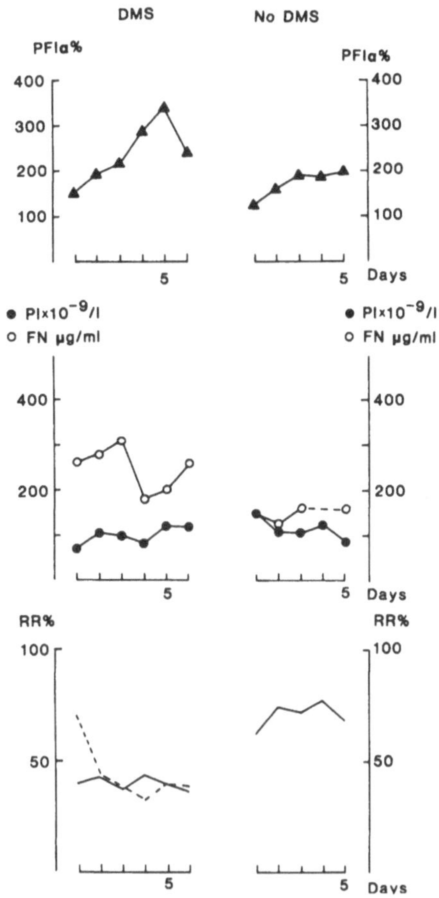


Figure 3.

Variation of mean values of different variables in 10 patients with a risk of developing the delayed microembolism syndrome (DMS). The five patients to the left developed DMS, whereas the five to the right did not. $PFI_a$ = primary fibrinolysis inhibitor: alpha. Pl = platelets. FN = fibronectin. RR = respiratory ratio. The dashed curve of RR represents the mean values in patients who developed DMS during the observation period. Values of RR below 50 % indicate DMS.

These peptides have a short half-life in the circulation, which is probably due to rapid enzymatic degradation, e.g. by angiotensin-converting enzyme and carboxypeptidase, and intravenous infusion of low molecular weight fibrin degradation products alone did not increase the vascular permeability in the lungs. However, when these products were infused together with a small dose of thrombin and a fibrinolysis inhibitor the lung weight was heavily increased (32).

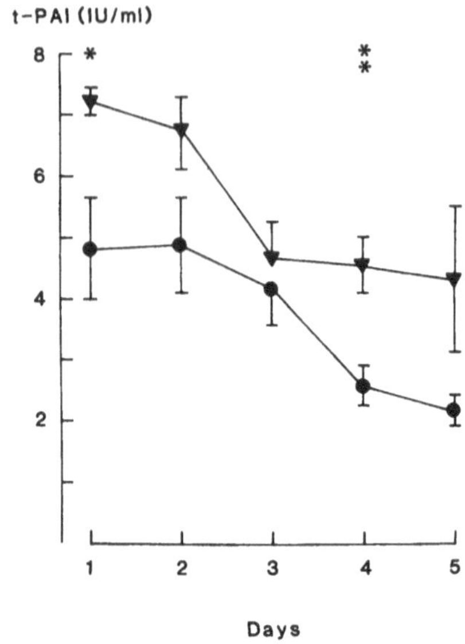


Figure 4.

The inhibitor against tissue plasminogen activator (t-PAI) in plasma in patients. For details see text to figure 3. ▼ = DMS ● = No DMS. X ± SE. * $p < 0.05$ ** $p < 0.01$.

In addition, when we injected peptide 6D subpleurally into the dog lung, this resulted in severe pulmonary edema (30). Injection of peptides 6A and 6D into the cat trachea has been found to cause an increased leakage of protein from the vessels (26), and inhalation of peptide 6A by guinea pigs led to an increased permeability to protein in the lungs (26). The same difference between local and systematic administration also seems to be true for other vaso-active substances such as histamine and bradykinin. Thus, although local administration of bradykinin results in edema, intravenous injection of massive doses of bradykinin does not result in an increase in macromolecular permeability.

When the fibrinolytic system functions normally, fibrin and fibrin degradation products leave the lungs rapidly and do not cause any damage to the pulmonary endothelium. If the fibrinolytic system is inhibited, and if the fibrinolytic activity in the circulating blood is reduced, fibrin remains in the lungs for a long time, resulting in local release of products from its degradation under the influence of local plasminogen activators and other proteases in the lungs, such as elastase. The fibrin passes between the endothelial cells into the extravascular tissue, where clearance of the previously mentioned peptides is much slower than slower than intravascularly. In patients, fibrin has been found between endothelial cells; these cells show dilated junctional gaps containing fibrin, and the cytoplasm in association with these junctions is dense and granular (45), indicating that fibrin and fibrin metabolites play a role in the induction of cellular damage. These changes seem to be specific for the delayed microembolism syndrome and have not been observed in other conditions. The same changes are seen in humans and dogs with this syndrome, indicating a common pathogenesis. When the fibrinolytic system is very strongly inhibited, an effect which has been induced in sheep by injection of tranexamic acid, the permeability is decreased (40), possibly as a result of greatly suppressed local release of fibrin degradation products.

Fibrinogen fragment -D may also participate in the development of the pulmonary injury, since infusion of this fragment into rabbits results in increased pulmonary microvascular permeability (43).

Terbutaline and isoprenaline, which are known to counteract cell contraction, inhibit the permeability-increasing effect of fibrin degradation products (29), which may suggest that these products can cause contraction of endothelial cells.

We have isolated two peptides (called 6A and 6D) obtained by plasmin degradation of human fibrin or fibrinogen that increase microvascular permeability, and one elastase degradation product Bβ 30-43, from fibrin or fibrinogen, with a stronger effect (Table I). Peptide 6A corresponds to residues 43-47 of the Bβ-chain and the undecapeptide 6D to residues 220-230 of the Aα-chain. Peptide Bβ 30-43 corresponds to residues 30-43 of the Bβ-chain of the fibrinogen.

| | |
|---|---|
| Peptide 6A | Ala-Arg-Pro-Ala-Lys |
| Peptide 6D | Ser-Gln-Leu-Gln-Lys-Val-Pro-<br>Pro-Gly-Trp-Lys |
| Peptide Bβ 30-43 | Arg-Pro-Ala-Pro-Pro-Pro-Ile-<br>Ser-Gly-Gly-Gly-Tyr-Arg-Ala |

Table I. Sequences of the fibrin(ogen) derived vasoactive peptides.

These peptides release histamine from mast cells, Bβ 30-43 being most potent (Fig. 5) (61).

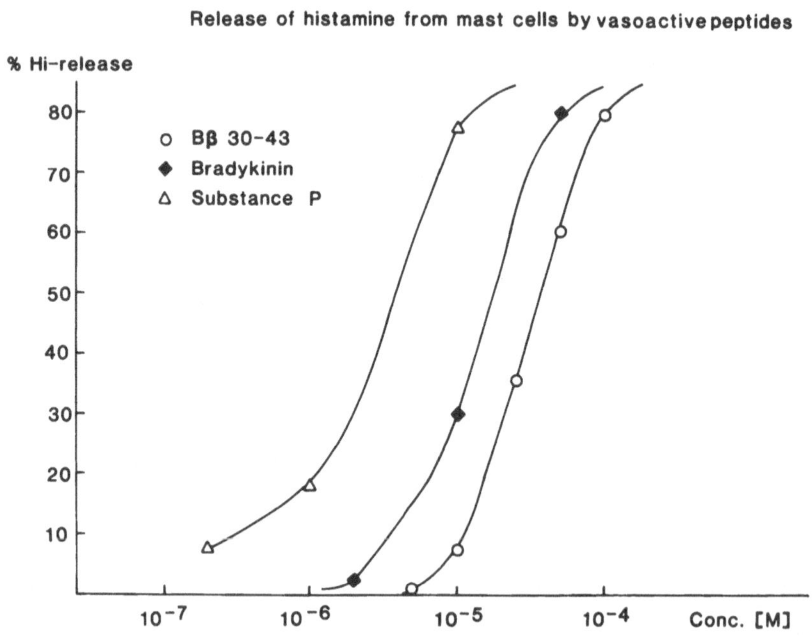


Figure 5.
Release of histamine (% Hi-release) from mast cells by vasoactive peptides.

The fact that most of their action on microvascular permeability can be inhibited by the $H_1$ blocker mepyramine maleate (Fig. 6) (61), indicates that histamine is a major mediator of their effect.

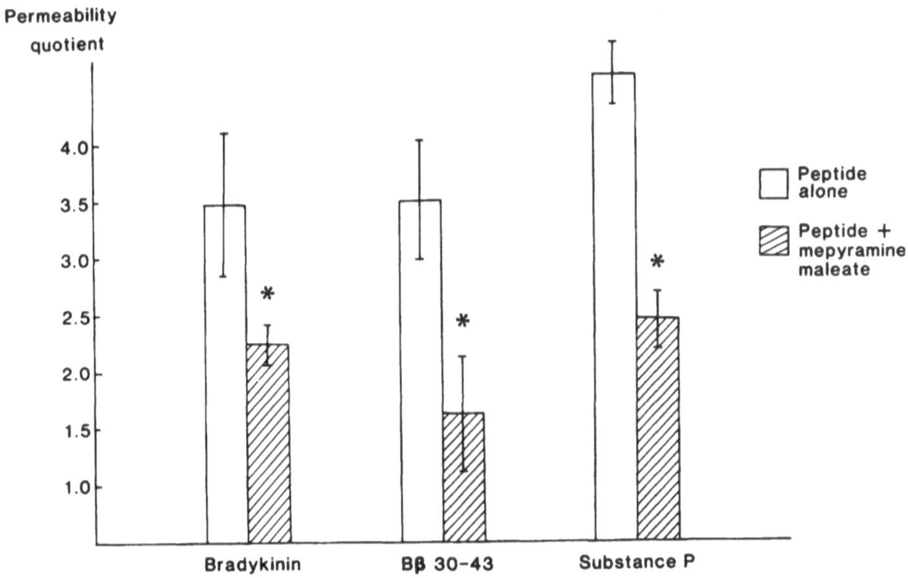


Figure 6.

The influence of 1 μg of mepyramine maleate per spot on the permeability-increasing effects of peptides in rat skin after intracutaneous injection, as expressed by the permeability quotient. Injected amounts: Bradykinin 2 μmol/spot, Bβ 30-43 5μmol/spot and substance P 1 μmol/spot.

The ability of the peptide Bβ 30-43 to release histamine may be attributable to the two basic amino acids, several prolines (Pro) and the aromatic acid tyrosine at the C-terminal part of the molecule. Basic amino acids as well as Pro residues and aromatic acids at the C-terminal end have been shown to be of significance for the release of histamine. It has also been demonstrated that an arginine (Arg) at the N-terminal end is important for the release of histamine and it is of interest to note that peptide Bβ 30-43, bradykinin and substance P all have an Arg at this position.

Peptide Bβ 30-43 shows certain similarities to bradykinin, with an Arg close to the N-terminal end, and several Pro and aromatic amino acids at the C-terminal part. The reason why bradykinin is somewhat more potent than Bβ 30-43 might possibly be that it contains two aromatic amino acids.

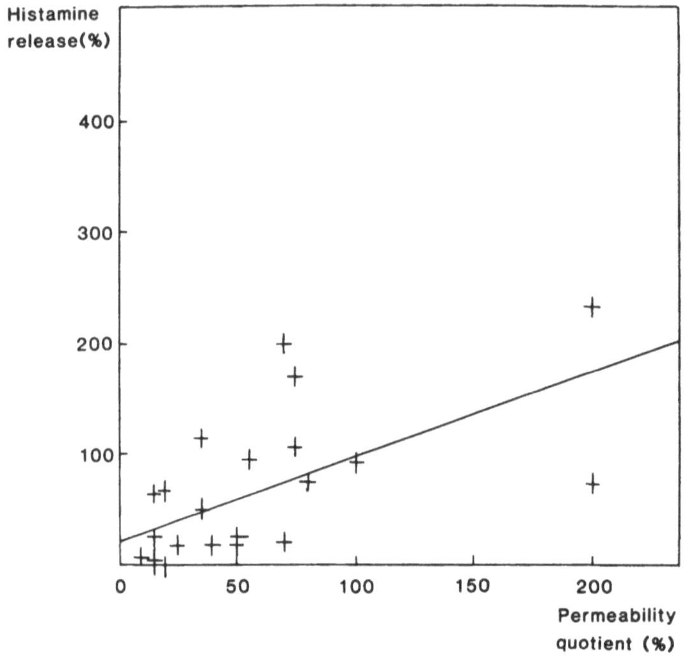


Figure 7.

Correlation between histamine release and permeability quotients for various analogues of peptide 6A. See text.

Fig. 7 illustrates the correlation between histamine release from rat mast cells and the increase in permeability to peptide 6A and to 32 analogues of this peptide in rat skin; the correlation coefficient was 0.4 x (62). Two peptides, Arg-Pro-Lys-Lys and Ala-Arg-Pro-Lys-Lys, had a very strong histamine-releasing capacity and were four times more potent than peptide 6A. Four peptides (Ala-Lys-Pro-Ala-Arg, Ala-Arg-Pro-Ala-Arg, Ala-Arg-Pro-Ala-D-Lys and Ala-Arg-Pro-Ala-D-Lys $(NH_2)$) had a very low capacity to release histamine in comparison with their ability to increase microvascular permeability in rat skin. Both analogues which were potent in releasing histamine, mentioned above, thus had the C-terminal sequence Lys-Lys and it is well known that peptides with a basic charge are potent releasers of histamine. The reason for the weaker effect of these analogues on microvascular permeability may lie in their enzymatic degradation in vivo, as a coboxypeptidase inhibitor strongly increased their effect on permeability (62). A lower capacity of carboxypeptidase for in vivo degradation might be one explanation for the finding that the four peptides with the C-terminal sequences Arg, Arg, D-Lys and D-Lys ($NH_2$), respectively, rather than L-Lys, had a more potent effect on microvascular permeability than could be expected from their histamine-releasing action, as the carboxypeptidase inhibitor seemed to have less effect on these peptides.

Pretreatment with indomethacin reduced the permeability-increasing effect of the peptides (62) (Table II), suggesting that in addition to histamine an arachidonic acid product might also be involved in the permeability increase. The effect of indomethacin should not be due to less release of histamine, as indomethacin did not diminish the 6A-induced

| | Permeability quotient |
|---|---|
| 6A | 4.1 ± 0.4 |
| Indo + 6A | 2.9 ± 0.3 X |
| 6A + mepyramine | 1.5 ± 0.4 X |
| Indo + 6A + mepyramine | 1.4 ± 0.3 X |

Table II. Effect of intravenously injected indomethacin (Indo) (4 mg/kg) on the permeability increasing effect of 6A in rats treated or non-treated with mepyramine maleate (mepyramine) (1 μg/spot), (n = 4). X = significantly different from 6A alone.

release of histamine from mast cells (62). Peptide 6A caused dilation of bovine mesenteric arteries both on direct application and when applied on preconstricted vessels (Fig. 8) (2). The peptide-induced relaxation was associated with a significant increase in cyclic AMP in the vessels (2). Application of this peptide resulted in an increase in the release of 6-keto-$PGF_{1\alpha}$ by the arteries. Pretreatment with indomethacin ($10^{-5}$) abolished the effects of 6A on the vessel tone, on the cyclic AMP content and on the release of 6-keto-$PGF_{1\alpha}$ (Fig. 9). Since peptide 6A induced release of prostacyclin from the vessels and indomethacin abolished the vasodilatory effect of this peptide, it is probable that the latter effect of 6A is caused by prostacyclin. The increase in cyclic AMP may indicate the existence of specific receptors for 6A. However, as indomethacin abolished the increase in cyclic AMP, it seems more likely that this increase is secondary to the prostacyclin release. Prostacyclin is known to increase cyclic AMP in blood vessels (37). Peptide 6A did not alter the level of cyclic GMP. Interestingly, prostacyclin has also

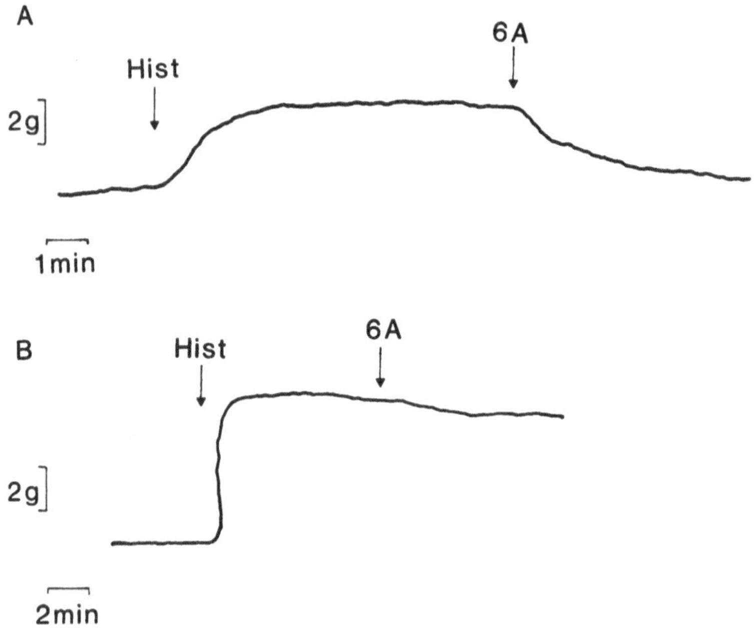


Figure 8.

Relaxant effect of peptide 6A (50 nmol/ml) in bovine mesenteric artery. The arteries were contracted by histamine (1 nmol/ml). In (B) the artery was preincubated with indomethacin (10 µmol/ml) for 20 minutes.

been reported not to change the level of cyclic GMP in blood vessels. Prostacyclin may potentiate the permeability enhancement due to histamine. The fact that indomethacin did not further decrease the permeability in rats treated with mepyramine maleate (Table II) indicates that prostacyclin alone does not increase permeability, but that it has to be combined with another mediator such as histamine.

Peptide 6A is an inhibitor of angiotensin converting enzyme ($I_{50}$ 1.9 x $10^{-5}$ M) (55). Peptide 6D has a much weaker inhibitory effect on this enzyme ($I_{50}$ 1.0 x $10^{-4}$ M) than 6A. A much lower concentration of this peptide, however, than of peptide 6A is required to induce histamine release from mast cells (25).

Inhibition of angiotensin converting enzyme might well be a contributory mechanism underlying the effect of peptide 6A on microvascular permeability. Of nine analogues that were more potent as inhibitors of angiotensin converting enzyme than peptide 6A itself, seven caused a stronger increase in vascular permeability than was expected from their histamine-releasing action (62). On the other hand, of 12 analogues that had a weaker inhibitory effect on this enzyme than peptide 6A, only one was more potent in increasing microvascular permeability than in inducing histamine release, and all the others were less potent. Peptides which more strongly inhibit angiotensin converting enzyme may be less rapidly degraded in vivo, and induce release of histamine over a longer period of time.

An increased plasma level of peptide 6A could possibly be one reason for the decreased activity of angiotensin converting enzyme observed in plasma of patients with ARDS (5, 20).

Low molecular weight fibrin degradation products are cytotoxic to endothelial cells, increase the release of $^{51}Cr$, decrease the uptake of $^{3}H$-adenine and decrease DNA synthesis in endothelial cells (13).

There are probably other additional mechanisms by which the fibrin trapped in the lungs can induce pulmonary damage. Thus,

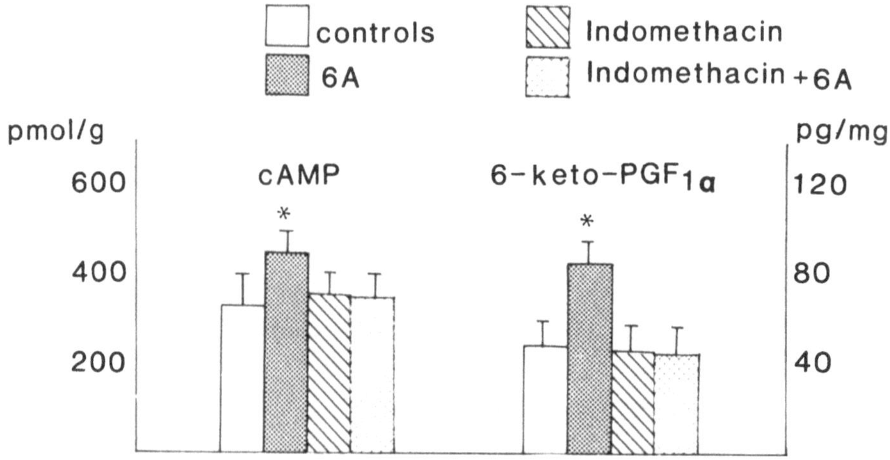


Figure 9.

Effects of peptide 6A (50 nmol/ml) on the cyclic AMP level and the release of prostacyclin in bovine mesenteric arteries. The arteries were incubated with peptide 6A for 5 minutes. Some arteries were preincubated with indomethacin (10 nmol/ml) for 20 minutes. Mean ± S.E.M. n = 4-6, * = significant increase compared with the other groups ($p < 0.01$).

tissue plasminogen activator and plasminogen are specifically adsorbed to the fibrin, resulting in local plasmin formation. Plasmin can activate the complement system, causing release of chemotactic factors such as $C5_a$. In addition, fibrin immobilizes leukocytes and may promote their contact with the vascular wall (40, 58). Depletion of leukocytes did not prevent the establishment of the severe permeability disturbance in our DMS model in the dog (11). This shows that the presence of leukocytes is not necessary for the development of the edema in this model, but does not rule out the possibility that these cells may contribute to the edema in other species, especially in patients with the delayed microembolism syndrome in whom infection or sepsis develops. Fibrin may enhance the trapping of leukocytes in the pulmonary vessels, and leukocytes release elastase, which in turn degrades fibrin, resulting in some peptides with a strong permeability-increasing capacity and also a chemotactic effect.

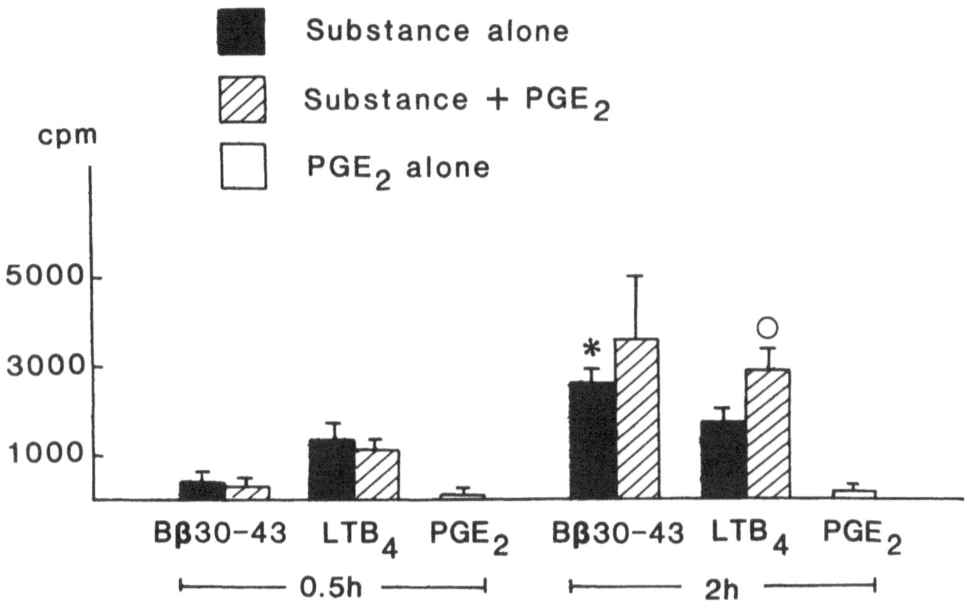


Figure 10

Effect of Bβ 30-43 (20 nmol), and $LTB_4$ (100 ng) alone or together with $PGE_2$ (1 µg) on polymorphonuclear emigration in rabbit skin. Mean ± S.E.M. n = 4. * Significantly different from Bβ at 0.5 h and from $LTB_4$ at 0.5 h and 2 h, ○ significantly different from $LTB_4$ alone at 2 h and from $LTB_4$+ $PGE_2$ at o.5 h.

Bβ 30-43 induces a significant increase in leukocyte emigration in rabbit skin (Fig 10.) (50). Addition of $PGE_2$ had no significant influence on the leukocyte accumulation due to peptide Bβ 30-43, but enhanced leukocyte emigration due to $LTB_4$, possibly by an increase in blood flow as a result of vasodilation, thus providing a larger vascular bed for leukocyte emigration. The reason why $PGE_2$ did not significantly enhance leukocyte emigration due to Bβ 30-43 might possibly be that this peptide induced release of the vasodilator $PGI_2$ and that further vasodilation by $PGE_2$ was not possible (Fig. 10) (50). Leukocyte products may also increase permeability by releasing oxygen-free radicals, lysosomal enzymes or leukotrienes. In granulocytopenic sheep, Brigham and coworkers (9, 10) found that the increase in lung permeability induced by endotoxin was diminished. The pulmonary damage in the delayed microembolism syndrome in the rat has also been reduced in animals made leukocytopenic by injection of anti-leukocytic serum (57). In sheep pretreated with superoxide dismutase-Ficoll the increase in pulmonary lymph flow caused by thrombin was blunted but not completely inhibited (41). The generation of superoxide anions may therefore play a role in the development of increased vascular permeability associated with pulmonary microembolism. The protective effect of superoxide dismutase may be due to removal of superoxide anions and to the subsequent lack of formation of hydroxyl radicals (41).

There seems to be an association between pulmonary edema, thromboxane production and leukocyte sequestration in the lungs. This has been suggested, for example, in studies with acid aspiration in the dog, in which model the cyclo-oxygenase inhibitor ibuprofen reduced thromboxane synthesis, leukocyte entrapment in the lungs and pulmonary edema (59). Thromboxane $A_2$ may be produced by the entrapped leukocytes and this prostanoid may activate other white cells to produce, for example, leukotrienes. Thromboxane is also known to augment leukocyte adhesiveness (60). Agglutinated leukocytes in the pulmonary microcirculation may damage endothelial cells in a manner which stimulates them to synthesize thromboxane (42). Although platelets are the main source of thromboxane in the blood in most species, leukocytes seem to be the main producers of thromboxane in inflammation (35). It is also of interest that aspirin seems to be more potent in inhibiting thromboxane production in the blood than in inflammatory exudates (35). These findings suggest that the leukocytes have to be stimulated in some way in order to produce thromboxane and that "low dose aspirin", although effective in reducing thromboxane production in the blood, may be less able to inhibit thromboxane production in tissues in pathological conditions.

Recent studies in humans and animals have shown that severe gas exchange disturbances may occur at a time when the water content of the lung is only modestly elevated. This might suggest that the role of pulmonary edema in the pathogenesis of the pulmonary dysfunction has been overestimated and that more attention should be directed towards shunting and airway disturbances.

Up to now diagnosis of the delayed microembolism syndrome is mainly based upon a progressive decrease in $pO_2$ which cannot be explained by other pulmonary disturbances such as pulmonary edema due to fluid overload or left heart failure, aspiration, pneumonia, atelectases or pulmonary contusion, and which is combined with the following: a low platelet count; an increase in factor VIII-related antigen (47) (Fig. 11); and a disturbance of the fibrinolytic system - the latter with an increase in primary fibrinolysis inhibitor: alpha and in the inhibitor against tissue plasminogen activator at an early stage, a decrease in plasminogen and, at a later stage, an increase in fibrin split products (34).

Altered circulating factor VIII complexes have been found in patients with acute respiratory failure and since they are produced and released by endothelial cells they have been considered sensitive indicators of pulmonary injury (19).

The appearance of the pulmonary radiograph is unspecific in the earlier stages, and early ventilator treatment with PEEP counteracts the classical radiographic pattern of bilateral alveolar densities characteristic of the delayed microembolism syndrome. Recently, serial pulmonary angiography has been tried in rats. In normal rats an arterial, a capillary and a venous phase could be identified. The capillary phase was characterized by homogeneous opacification of the lung parenchyma, resulting in a structureless appearance. In rats with early stages of the delayed microembolism syndrome there is non-homogeneous opacification of the lung parenchyma in the capillary phase, suggesting large regional differences in capillary perfusion (64). Some areas may lack capillary circulation, while others may display increased perfusion. No change in the circulation time through the lungs was noted at videodensitometry, which may be explained by arteriovenous shunting. This shunting may partly explain the lack of oxygenation. Hypoxemia may therefore be caused not only by a decrease in the ventilation/perfusion ratio due, for example to perfusion of alveoli filled with fluid, but also to right-left intrapulmonary shunts.

| Day | 1 | 2 | 3 | 4 | 5 |
|---|---|---|---|---|---|
| All patients | 163±78 (13) | 154±65 (18) | 159±56 (14) | 170±41 (12) | 182±51 (11) |
| DMS | 196±78 (6) | 206±52 (7) | 197±53 (7) | 208±16 (6) | 222±20 (6) |
| Non-DMS | 135±64 (7) | 121±50 (11) | 120±25 (7) | 132±15 (6) | 135±33 (5) |
| Significance | | ** | ** | *** | *** |

Figure 11.

Factor VIII-related antigen (percent of normal human plasma; mean ± S.D.) on days 1-5 after trauma or sepsis in 19 patients at risk, of whom 8 developed the delayed microembolism syndrome (DMS) and 11 did not. Number of patients within brackets. Day 1 is the first day of investigation in the Intensive Care Unit. In every patient the traumatic or septic event had occurred 2-12 h before the start of the investigation schedule.

Thus pulmonary angiography can add further diagnostic information in patients suffering from this syndrome. Recently pulmonary angiography performed in a large number of these patients revealed filling defects in small vessels in most of them (33).

During recent years, a gratifying decrease in the number of deaths from delayed microembolism has been noted (Fig. 12). The incidence of the delayed microembolism syndrome in our district (one million inhabitants) is about 60 per year, and the death rate from this syndrome has now decreased to less than 5 percent. This reduction is probably due to improvements in prophylaxis and therapy. For prophylaxis, 500 ml of dextran 70 has been administered daily during the first days after trauma. Infusion of dextran has been found to greatly decrease the capacity for inhibition of fibrinolysis in

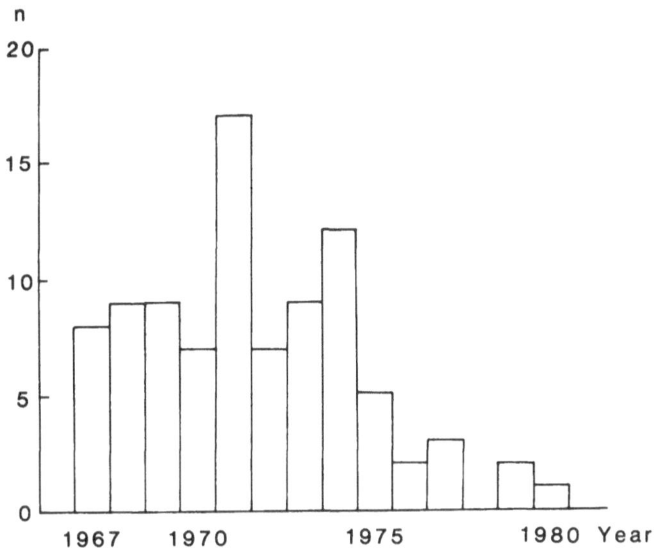


Figure 12.

Number of deaths from the delayed microembolism syndrome recorded at our department yearly from 1967 - 1980. Note the decrease in recent years.

patients (15), an effect which seems to be due to alteration of the fibrin network (14). This fibrin has an increased ability to bind plasmin, whereby the plasmin is better protected from the efficient primary fibrinolysis inhibitor $\alpha_2$-antiplasmin.

Therapeutically, heparin treatment to the upper normal value for activated thromboplastin time has probably contributed to the results. Because of the danger of bleeding, heparin is never administered to patients with brain injury or pelvic fractures.

Low molecular weight fragments of heparin carry a lower risk of bleeding and have recently been tried in animals. They should be very interesting in the prophylaxis and treatment of these patients in the future.

The effects of other substances on the delayed microembolism syndrome have been investigated in animal experiments. Brinase (a protease from Aspergillus oryzae) is a substance used in lysis of occluded external hemodialysis shunts, arterial thrombi, and non-recent peripheral arterial obstruction. Treatment with brinase has been found to result in greatly improved elimination of fibrin from the lungs in rats with induced intravascular coagulation (23). The coagulation-induced pulmonary damage was also reduced.

Intravenously infused tissue plasminogen activator accelerates the elimination of fibrin in rats (18), whereas synthetic fibrinolysis inhibitors (53) and the primary fibrinolysis inhibitor ($\alpha_2$-antiplasmin) (16), infused intravenously, greatly decrease the elimination of fibrin, with pulmonary damage as a result. Tissue plasminogen activator may prove to be an interesting drug for these patients in the future.

Trasylol reduces the pulmonary trapping of fibrin in rats following induction of coagulation by thromboplastin (22). Trasylol (aprotinin) delays the elimination of fibrin from the lungs in normal animals, but has no effect on the elimination in animals with an inhibited fibrinolytic system.

Treatment with alpha-receptor blockers has been used in many patients with post-traumatic shock. A reduced flood flow in the pulmonary capillaries and greatly delayed elimination of fibrin have been found in animals given the alpha-receptor - blocking agent phenoxybenzamine (31). Infusion of albumin counteracted the effect of this agent. The therapeutic advantage of alpha-receptor blockade might thus be lost by the hazards related to impeded elimination of fibrin, and the results stress the importance of adequate volume replacement.

In rat experiments inhibitors of the angiotensin converting enzyme have been shown to diminish the pulmonary edema and the reduction in $pO_2$ due to microembolism. These effects may be attributable to a decreased pulmonary arterial pressure.

Corticosteroids are frequently used in some hospitals in patients with the delayed microembolism syndrome, e.g. methylprednisolone in a dose of 1-2 g/day in the initial stage. Administration of hydrocortisone in rats results in delayed elimination of fibrin (24), seemingly due to an inhibitory effect of this substance on inhibition of the fibrinolytic system. Administration of hydrocortisone leads to increased mobilization of free fatty acids from adipose tissue, which may stimulate the synthesis of $\alpha_2$-antiplasmin in the liver. In addition, corticosteroids may enhance shunting by interfering with normal hypoxic vasoconstriction in areas of poor ventilation or edema, and may adversely affect leukocyte function, thus lowering the resistance to infection.

However, corticosteroids also have beneficial effects. Thus, it has been shown both in animals and patients with septic shock that methylprednisolone given in a dose of 30 mg/kg every 6 h can significantly reduce edema in the lungs when administrered at an early stage (8), suggesting that one mechanism may be an inhibition of phospolipase $A_2$ with decreased activation of the archidonic acid cascade.

As yet there have been no controlled clinical studies on cyclo-oxygenase and thromboxane-synthetase inhibitors, but results from animal experiments show that these drugs have a beneficial effect in the early phases of the syndrome, which is due to inhibition of thromboxane synthesis, but a less good effect - sometimes with an increase in the edema - in later phases, possibly due to enhancement of blood flow to damaged capillaries.

Recently exchange transfusion or combined plasmapheresis and leukopheresis has been tried in patients with shock lung due to sepsis. With this therapy a number of products of the various cascade systems are removed.

<u>To sum up</u>, fibrin has been found in the lungs of all patients with idiophathic acute respiratory distress. Clinical and autopsy studies have shown an association between fibrin in the lungs and respiratory distress after trauma. Prophylaxis and treatment with the aim of decreasing the fibrin deposition in the lungs, e.g. with dextran and heparin, have been associated with a considerable reduction of the death rate from acute respiratory distress after trauma in our region, whereas the overall incidence of and death rate in ARDS internationally do not seem to have decreased.

Mechanical blockage of the vessels does not seem to be a major mechanism underlying the effect of the fibrin. This fibrin is an enormous substrate for local release of potent vasoactive substances, some of which originate from the fibrin itself and others, especially in patients with complicating sepsis, from leukocytes trapped in the fibrin network. Many observations indicate that several other mediators such as products of the arachidonic acid cascade and the complement system, as well as histamine and bradykinin, can modulate the outcome of the disease and that the importance of the different mediators varies with the stage of the disease. It should be borne in mind, however, that most of our knowledge in this field derives from animal experiments and can only be extra-polated to the clinical situation with caution.

REFERENCES


1. Andersson P, Brange C, Saldeen K, Saldeen T. Fibrin(ogen) derived vasoactive peptides release thromboxane, prostacyclin and histamine in isolated, perfused guinea-pig lung. Thromb. Res. Manuscript.

2. Andersson RGC, Saldeen K, Saldeen T. A fibrin(ogen) derived pentapeptide induces vasodilation, prostacyclin release and an increase in cyclic AMP. Thromb Res. 1983; 30:213-218.

3. Bagge L, Saldeen T. The primary fibrinolysis inhibitor and trauma. Thromb Res 1978; 13:1131-1136.

4. Bagge L, Hedstrand U, Höök M, Johansson S, Lind E, Modig J, Saldeen T. Fibrinolysis inhibition and fibrinectin in the blood in patients with the delayed microembolism syndrome. Ups J Med Sci 1983; 88:81-94.

5. Bedrossian C W, Woo J, Miller W C et al. Decreased angiotensin converting enzyme in adult respiratory distress syndrome. Am. J. Clin. Pathol. 1978; 70:244-247.

6. Belew M, Gerdin B, Porath J, Saldeen T. Isolation of vasoactive peptides from human fibrin and fibrinogen degraded by plasmin. Thromb Res 1978; 13:983-994.

7. Blaisdell, FW. Respiratory insufficiency syndrome. Clinical and pathological definition. J. Trauma 1973; 13:195.

8. Brigham KL, Bowers RE, McKeen CR. Methylprednisolone prevention of increased lung vascular permeability following endotoxemia in sheep. J. Clin. Invest. 1981; 67:1103-1110.

9. Brigham KL. Mechanisms of lung injury. In: Bone RC, ed. Clinics in Chest Medicine. Philadelphia, WB Saunders, 1982; 9-24.

10. Brigham KL, Lloyd JE, Newman JH et al. Granulocytes in acute lung vascular injury in unanaesthetized sheep. Chest 1982; 81:56S-57S.

11. Busch C, Lindquist O, Saldeen T. Respiratory insufficiency in the dog induced by pulmonary microembolism and inhibition of fibrinolysis. Effect of defibrinogenation, leucopenia and thrombocytopenia. Acta Chir. Scand. 1974; 140:255-266.

12. Busch C, Dahlgren S, Jakobson S, Jung B, Modig J, Saldeen T. The use of $^{125}$I-labelled fibrinogen for determination of fibrin trapping in the lungs in patients developing the microembolism syndrome. Acta Anaesthisiol Scand Suppl 1975; 57:46-54.

13. Busch C, Gerdin B. Effect of low molecular weight fibrin degradation products on endothelial cells in culture. Thromb. Res. 1981; 22:33-39.

14. Carlin G, Saldeen T. Influence of dextran 70 on the action of the primary fibrinolysis inhibitor ($\alpha_2$-plasmin inhibitor). Thromb Res 1978; 12:681-686.

15. Carlin G, Saldeen T. Effect of dextran on fibrinolysis inhibition activity in serum. Thromb Res 1978; 12:1165-1175.

16. Carlin G, Einarsson M, Saldeen T. Delayed elimination of fibrin from the lungs in rats given $\alpha_2$-antiplasmin. Thromb Haemost 1981; 46:757-758.

17. Carlin G, Saldeen T. Studies on posttraumatic fibrinolysis inhibition by use of tissue plasminogen activator. Haemostasis 1982; 11:85.

18. Carlin G, Einarsson M, Saldeen T. Tissue plasminogen activator effectively lyses intravascular fibrin deposits in the rat lung. Progress in Fibrinolysis VI. Churchill Livingstone 1983; pp 471-474.

19. Carvalho ACA, Bellman SM, Saullo VJ, Zapol WM. Altered factor VIII in acute respiratory failure. N Engl J Med 1982; 307:1113-1119.

20. Casey L, Krieger B, Kohler J et al: Decreased serum angiotensin converting enzyme in adult respiratory distress syndrome with sepsis. Crit Care Med 1981; 9:651-654.

21. Connors AF, McCaffree DR, Rogers RM. The adult respiratory distress syndrome. D M 1981; 27:1-75.

22. Diffang C, Saldeen T. Effect of Trasylol on fibrin deposition and elimination in the lungs of rats with intravascular coagulation induced by thrombin or thromboplastin. Thromb Res 1974; 5:263-276.

23. Diffang C, Saldeen T. Effect of brinase (protease I from Aspergillus oryzae) on the elimination of fibrin from the lungs and pulmonary damage in rats with induced intravascular coagulation and inhibited fibrinolysis. Throm Res 1976; 9:611-622.

24. Diffang C, Saldeen T. Effect of hydrocortisone on the elimination of fibrin from the pulmonary vessels in the rat. Thromb Res 1978; 13: 2536.

25. Eriksson M, Saldeen K, Saldeen T, Strandberg K, Wallin R. Fibrin-derived vasoactive peptides release histamine. Int J Microcirc Clin Exp 1983; 2:337-345.

26. Erjefält I, Persson C, Saldeen T. Framkallande lungödem med substanser med kort halveringstid i blod. Läkarsällskapets Riksstämma, Stockholm 1981, p. 497. Abstr. (Swe.)

27. Fowler AA, Walchat S, Giclas PC et al. Chest 1982; 81: (suppl) 50S-51S.

28. Fowler AA, Baird M, Eberle D et al. Attack-rates and mortality of the adult respiratory distress syndrome in patients with predisposition. Am. Rev. Respir. Dis. 1983; 125:77.

29. Gerdin B, Saldeen T. Effect of fibrin degradation products on microvascular permeability. Thromb. Res. 1978; 13:995-1006.

30. Gerdin B, Belew M, Lindquist O, Saldeen T. Effect of a fibrin derived peptide on pulmonary microvascular permeability. In: Saldeen T, ed. The Microembolism Syndrome. Almqvist & Wiksell International. Stockholm 1979; pp. 233-239.

31. Gerdin B, Diffang C, Saldeen T. Effect of α-receptor blockade on the rate of fibrin elimination from the rat lung. Circ. Shock 1980; 7:93-101.

32. Gerdin B, Diffang C, Saldeen T. Pulmonary insufficiency in the rat after intravascular coagulation and inhibition of fibrinolysis. I. Studies on some pathogenetic mechanisms. Eur Surg Res 1981; 13:402-413.

33. Greene R, Zapol WM, Snider MT, Reid C, Snow R, O´Connell RS, Novelline RA. Early bedside detection of pulmonary vascular occlusion during acute respiratory failure. Am Rev Respir Dis 1981; 124:593-601.

34. Haynes JB, Hyers TM, Gicleas PC et al. Elevated fibrin-(ogen) degradation products in adult respiratory distress syndrome. Am. Rev. Respir. Dis. 1980; 122: 841-847.

35. Higgs GA, Moncadaa S, Salmon JA, Seager K. The source of thromboxane and prostaglandings in experimental inflammation. Br. J. Pharmac. 1983; 79:863-868.

36. Högstorp H, Saldeen T. Synthesis of $\alpha_2$-antiplasmin by rat liver cells. Thromb Res 1982; 28:19-25.

37. Ito T, Ogawa K, Enomoto I, Hashimoto H, Kai I, Satake T. Comparison of the effects of $PGI_2$ and $PGE_1$ on coronary and systemic hemodynamics and coronary arterial cyclic nucleotide levels in dogs. Advances in Prostaglandin and Thromboxane Research 1980; 7:641-646.

38. Kruithof EKO, Ransijn A, Bachmann F. Inhibition of tissue plasminogen activator by human plasma. Progress in Fibrinolysis 1983; VI: 365-369.

39. Lee CT, Fein AM, Lippman M, et al. Elastolytic activity in pulmonary lavage fluid from patient with adult respiratory distress syndrome. N Engl J Med 1981; 304:192-196.

40. Malik AB. Pulmonary microembolism. Physiological Reviews 1983; 63:1114-1207.

41. Malik AB, Fenton II JW, Johnson A, Cooper J, Bizios R, Minnear FL. Trombin-induced pulmonary micro-embolism mechanisms of lung vascular injury. In this volume.

42. McDonald JWD, Morgon MAE, Townsend ER, Cooper JD. Thromboxane synthesis by sources other than platelets in association with complement-induced pulmonary leukostasis and pulmonary hypertension in sheep. Circulation Research 1983; 82:1-6.

43. Manwaring D, Thorning D, Curreri PW. Mechanism of acute pulmonary dysfunction induced by fibrinogen degradation product D. Surgery 1978; 84:45-54.

44. McGuire WW, Spragg RG, Cohen AB, et al. Studies on the pathogenesis of the adult respiratory distress syndrome. J. Clin Invest 1982; 69:543-553.

45. MoCostabella P, Lindquist O, Kapanci Y, Saldeen T. Increased vascular permeability in the delayed microembolism syndrome. Experimental and human finding. Microvasc Res 1978; 15:275-286.

46. Modig J, Busch C, Olerud S, Saldeen T, Waernbaum G. Arterial hypotension and hypoxaemia during total hip replacement: the importance of thromboplastic products, fat embolism and acrylic monomers. Acta Anaesthesiol Scand 1975; 19: 28-43.

47. Modig J, Borg T, Wegenius G, Bagge L, Saldeen T. The value of variables of disseminated intravascular coagulation in the diagnosis of adult respiratory distress syndrome. Acta Anaesthesiol Scand 1983; 27:369-375.

48. Murray JF: Mechanisms of acute respiratory failure. Am. Rev. Respir. Dis. 1977; 1071:115-122.

49. Saba TM, Blumenstock FA, Scovill WA, Bernard H. Cryoprecipitate reversal of opsonic $\alpha_2$ surface binding glycoprotein deficiency in septic surgical and trauma patients. Science 1978; 201:622-624.

50. Saldeen K, Christie N, Nelson WR, Movat HZ. Effect of a fibrin(ogen) derived vasoactive peptide on polymorphonuclear leukocyte emigration. Thromb. Res. In press.

51. Saldeen P, Saldeen T. Increased synthesis of thromboxane in atheromatous vessels. Thromb Res 1983; 31:591-597.

52. Saldeen P, Esquivel CO, Björck CG, Bergqvist D, Saldeen T. Thromboxane production in umbilical vein grafts. Thromb Res 1984; 33:259-267.

53. Saldeen T. Quantitative determination of intravascular coagulation in the lungs of experimental animals. Scand J Haematol 1969; 6: 205-215.

54. Saldeen T. The microembolism syndrome. Microvasc Res 1976; 11:227-259.

55. Saldeen T, Ryan JW, Berryer P. A peptide derived from fibrin(ogen) inhibits angiotensin converting enzyme and potentiated the effects of bradykinin. Thromb Res 1981; 23:465-470.

56. Sandler H. Saldeen T. Effect of nicotinic acid on the amount of fibrin in the posttraumatic rat lung. Thromb Res 1979; 15:703.

57. Sandler H, Saldeen T. Effect of an inhibitor of thromboxane synthesis (UK-37, 248-01) on thrombin-induced pulmonary insufficiency in the rat. Thromb Haemost 1981; 46:279.

58. Shaw JO, Henson PM, Henson J, Webster RO. Lab Invest 1980; 42;547-558.

59. Utsunomiya T, Krausz MM, Valeri CR, Shepro D, Hechtman H.B. Treatment of aspiration pneumonia with ibuprofen and prostacyclin. Surgery 1981; 90:170-176.

60. Spagnuolo PJ, Ellner JJ, Hassid A, Thromboxane $A_2$ mediates augumented polymorphonuclear leukocyte adhesiveness. J Clin Invest 1980; 66:406-414.

61. Wallin R, Saldeen K, Belew M, Ohlsson K, Saldeen T. Purification and characteristics of a vasoactive peptide derived from elastase degradation of human fibrin(ogen). Fibrinogen-Structure, Function. In press.

62. Wallin R, Saldeen K, Saldeen T. Structure-function studies on a vasoactive pentapeptide derived form plasmin degradation of human fibrin(ogen). Fibrinogen-Structure, Function. In press.

63. Wallin R, Belew M, Ohlsson K, Saldeen T. Purification of vaso-active peptides from human fibrinogen degraded by hyman leucocyte elastase. Thromb Haemost 1981; 46:52.

64. Wegener T, Wegenius G, Saldeen T, Eriksson U. Serial pulmonary angiography in rats with pulmonary damage due to intravascular coagulation. Acta Radiol Diag 1983; 24:449-457.

FSC
www.fsc.org
MIX
Papier | Fördert
gute Waldnutzung
FSC® C083411

Zeitfracht Medien GmbH
Ferdinand-Jühlke-Straße 7
99095 Erfurt, Deutschland
produktsicherheit@kolibri360.de